HEALTH AND HEALTH BEHAVIOR AMONG ELDERLY AMERICANS:
AN AGE-STRATIFICATION PERSPECTIVE

Fredric D. Wolinsky, Ph.D., is Professor of Medicine in the Division of General Internal Medicine of the Department of Medicine, at the Indiana University School of Medicine. His principal responsibilities there involve the continuation of his longstanding research program on the use of health services by older Americans. Funded by a prestigious MERIT award from the National Institute on Aging, this research focuses on the developmental course of health and health behavior among the elderly. Using panel data from the Longitudinal Study on Aging, Dr. Wolinsky is specifically addressing such thorny matters as the consistency of health services utilization over time, the interrelationships between the different dimensions of health services utilization, and the role of health services utilization in the risk for institutionalization and death.

Health and Health Behavior Among Elderly Americans:

An Age-Stratification Perspective

FREDRIC D. WOLINSKY

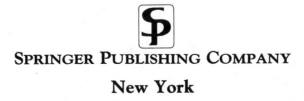

SPRINGER PUBLISHING COMPANY

New York

Springer Publishing Company, Inc.
536 Broadway
New York, NY 10012

90 91 92 93 94 / 5 4 3 2 1

Library of Congress Cataloging-in-Publication Data

Wolinsky, Fredric D.
    Health and health behavior among elderly Americans : an age-stratification perspective / Fredric D. Wolinsky.
        p. cm.
    Includes bibliographical references.
    ISBN 0-8261-7410-8
    1. Aged—Medical care—United States—Utilization.   2. Aged—Health and hygiene—United States.   3. Health behavior—United States—Age factors.   I. Title.
    RA408.A3W64   1990
    362.1′9897′00973—dc20   90-9417
                                                                          CIP

Printed in the United States of America

For MICHAEL COLLIN,
and the miracles of life.

Contents

Acknowledgments

This monograph would not have been possible without the continued support of several individuals and institutions. The research reported here was conducted between 1984 and 1989, during which time I was the recipient of a Research Career Development Award (RCDA) from the National Institute on Aging (K04-AG00328). Rod Coe served as my mentor, colleague, and friend from the time that the initial RCDA application was submitted to the completion of the last chapter. Indeed, although I left St. Louis University Medical Center in 1985, Rod graciously and effectively continued to be my principal adviser. This book and I are that much the better for it.

I have also benefited from the good will and stewardship of two individuals at the National Institute on Aging. Matilda Riley sought support for my RCDA from the beginning. Without her sponsorship, the award would never have been made. Similarly, Marcia Ory worked diligently at seeing that my research results were effectively communicated to appropriate audiences both at the institute, and elsewhere. Without Matilda's and Marcia's efforts, this study simply would not have been possible.

At one stage or another, this book and I have benefited greatly from the detailed comments and suggestions of three fine reviewers. Although I do not know if I have done justice to their recommendations, I am truly appreciative of the guidance provided by Larry Branch, Marie Haug, and Tom Wan. During the years I have been assisted on this project by several graduate students. For this help I wish to thank Connie Arnold, Kathy Dietrich, Lih-jiuan Fann, Ray Mosely, and Indira Nallapati. Finally, I wish to thank Lori Cheatham for producing camera-ready copy for the tables.

FREDRIC D. WOLINSKY
Indianapolis, Indiana

HEALTH AND HEALTH BEHAVIOR AMONG ELDERLY AMERICANS:
AN AGE-STRATIFICATION PERSPECTIVE

Chapter 1

Age-Stratification Perspective

The present interest in the patterns of health and health behavior exhibited by elderly Americans is motivated by two questions: What are these patterns, and what causes them? To be sure, these are not new queries. Indeed, as the reader shall see in Chapter 2, these issues have been under investigation for quite some time. Such familiar themes, however, are transformed into new challenges when viewed from the age-stratification perspective: Do the patterns of health and health behavior and their causes change as particular birth cohorts age, as they move through history, or as they are replaced by successive generations? Addressing these issues requires the use of longitudinal theory, methods, and data. These subjects are the focus of this book.

The purpose of this chapter is to introduce the reader to the longitudinal theory (i.e., the age-stratification perspective), and to the longitudinal methods (i.e., the techniques of cohort analysis) that logically flow from it. Accordingly, the present chapter contains two major sections. The first involves theoretical issues. It begins with a consideration of the fundamental building blocks of the age-stratification perspective. These are the concepts of aging (i.e., developmental), period (i.e., historical), and cohort (i.e., reference group identification based on years of birth) effects. After defining each concept at the biological, psychological, and social levels, illustrative examples related to the health and health behavior of elderly Americans are presented. The focus then shifts to the systematic integration and articulation of the aging, period, and cohort concepts under the umbrella of the age-stratification perspective. This includes discussions of the principles of aging and social change, the dynamic tension between them, and the asynchrony of their progression.

The second section of this chapter involves methodological issues. It presents the rudiments of the standard cohort analytic techniques that have been developed to permit the separation of age, period, and cohort effects in synthetic longitudinal studies. This includes the logic of cohort methods, the three major obstacles to interpreting standard cohort tables, and the techniques for visually inspecting them. A deceivingly simple example involving the public's interest in politics is used to illustrate the logic, utility, and complexity of cohort methods. The application of more sophisticated statistical techniques for the resolution of the identification problem is then discussed. The chapter concludes with a brief overview of what is to come in the remaining chapters of the book.

AGING, PERIOD, AND COHORT EFFECTS

Perhaps the easiest and most straightforward way to begin any discussion of the age-stratification perspective is to select an excerpt from the work of its principal figure, Matilda White Riley. In her 1986 Presidential Address to the American Sociological Association, Riley (1987) outlined the importance of this approach as follows:

> A sociology of age provides an analytical framework for understanding the interplay between human lives and changing social structures. Its mission is to examine the interdependence between (1) aging over the life course as a social process and (2) societies and groups as stratified by age, with the succession of cohorts as the link connecting the two. This special field of age draws on sociology as a whole and contributes to it through reformulation of traditional emphases on process and change, on the multiple interdependent levels of the system, and on the multidimensionality of sociological concerns as they touch on related aspects of other disciplines. (p. 1)

Thus, for Riley the age-stratification approach represents the systematic and multileveled examination of the iterative interaction between aging and social change (see also Glenn, 1976; Palmore, 1978).

In the complex process alluded to earlier, three different effects are at work: aging, period, and cohort. Each of these operates at the biological, psychological, and social levels to produce the observed social change. Therefore, to facilitate the presentation of the age-stratification perspective, age, period, and cohort effects must first be considered separately. Only then can the systematic framework be presented.

Aging Effects

Surprising as it may seem, definitions of aging are frequently absent from the work of gerontologists and geriatricians. More often than not a tacit assumption simply exists that the reader will understand what the author means by the phenomenon of aging. This aversion to defining aging, however, is not uniform across the levels at which such changes occur (see Birren & Cunningham, 1985). Biological scientists are the most likely to provide definitions of aging; psychological scientists do so only rarely; and social scientists hardly ever define what they mean by aging. As a result, it would appear that either (a) the relevance of aging as a variable (or at least the use of chronological age as its index) in the study of human behavior varies across these fields, or (b) the maturity of these fields in studying aging varies. On reflection, both seem plausible.

Biological definitions of aging focus on the growth, maturation, and senescence processes. Cowdry (1942) has written:

> Since almost all living organisms pass through a sequence of changes, characterized by growth, development, maturation and finally senescence, ageing presents a broad biological problem. (p. 15)

Thus, the focus of biological scientists appears to be on the length of life (or time to death) of organisms.

That length of life is thought to be determined by two processes. One involves involuntary cumulative effects that are typified by the inevitable modification and decline at the cellular level (frequently referred to as "programmed" or "endogenous" changes; see Cape, Coe, & Rossman, 1983). The other involves those effects resulting from trauma, disease, and impairment that alter cellular integrity (frequently referred to as "environmental" or "exogenous" changes; see Finch & Schneider, 1985). Biological scientists use chronological age as a marker for both processes. For the former it serves as a relatively straightforward developmental or staging index, with the (at least implicit) recognition of the heterogeneity of the senescence

process within species (see Comfort, 1956). For the latter it represents a much less straightforward index of the risk of exposure to
environmental hazards.

An example of biological aging is the consistent change, after
reaching maturity, of sleep patterns associated with the aging process.
Indeed, despite the paucity of longitudinal studies of sleep and aging,
Dement et al. (1985) have concluded that:

> certain tendencies seem well established. Advancing age is associated
> with increasing interruption of sleep, decreasing amount and per-
> centage of SWS [slow wave sleep], deterioration of circadian organi-
> zation, increasing prevalence of disordered breathing during sleep,
> and increasing prevalence of periodic leg movements. (p. 711–712)

These age-dependent changes (especially in the circadian rhythm)
have considerable relevance. Noting the striking relationship between
circadian disruption and depression among the nonelderly, Dement
et al. (1985) speculate that the remarkably higher rate of depression
among the elderly may be secondary to the greater prevalence of
circadian disruption among them. That would suggest interventions
be directed not at depression per se, but at the underlying cause (i.e.,
circadian disruption). Unfortunately, it is not yet clear whether these
observed age-dependent changes in sleep patterns are the result of
"normal" or "pathological" aging.

When psychological scientists define aging, they tend to take a tack
similar to that of the biologists. Indeed, the psychology of aging draws
heavily on the biomedical model (see Estes, 1988; Lyman, 1988). For
example, Birren and Renner (1977) define aging this way:

> Aging refers to the regular changes that occur in mature genetically
> representative organisms living under representative environmental
> conditions. (p. 4)

Their definition recognizes that aging effects may be either positive or
negative, and may occur at any point during the life-span, as long as
the changes are regular. Moreover, the scope conditions of this definition avoid rare genetic problems and the occurrence of atypical environmental conditions (see Birren & Cunningham, 1985). Thus, they
focus on "pure" or "normal" aging effects.

Perhaps the most important difference between the biological and
psychological approaches to studying aging lies in the use of chronological age as a marker. As indicated earlier, biological scientists
depend on chronological age as a direct measure of the aging process,
regardless of whether it represents an endogenous or exogenous ef-

fect. In contrast, psychological scientists use chronological age only as an indirect or proxy indicator of behavior whose changes are typically related to (but not dependent on) the passage of time. The crucial difference here involves the greater recognition of and emphasis on the heterogeneity of individual organisms by psychologists. They are more concerned with tracking ordered stages of development that are far more loosely associated with any chronological age markers.

An example of psychological aging involves the classic debate about the question of whether age-related changes in intelligence and cognition exist. The traditional view, supported primarily by cross-sectional studies and expressed here by Botwinick (1977), answered in the affirmative:

> after reviewing the available literature, both recent and old, the conclusion here is that decline in intellectual ability is clearly part of the aging picture. (p. 580)

Because of the more recent reports of Schaie and colleagues, however, based on data from the Seattle Longitudinal Study (see Schaie, 1981; Schaie & Hertzog, 1983, 1986; Schaie, Labouvie, & Buech, 1973) that traditional view has been softening.

Indeed, even Botwinick (1977) notes that these data have been very helpful in:

> bringing attention to what has been underemphasized in the older literature, via., these declines may start later in life than heretofore thought and they may be smaller in magnitude; they may also include fewer functions. (p. 580)

At the same time that the proponents of the traditional view have been softening, so have the views of Schaie and his colleagues. In particular, they now recognize the existence of age-related declines in intelligence and cognitive ability, but maintain that these declines generally do not begin until the fifth or sixth decade of life (see Labouvie-Vief, 1985).

Perhaps the most interesting aspect of this debate has been the increased focus on what accounts for individual differences in age-related changes in intelligence and cognition during the life course. Data from the Seattle Longitudinal Study have identified several factors that account for these differences. It seems that having cardiovascular and other chronic diseases (Hertzog, Schaie, & Gribbin, 1978), living in unfavorable environments related to low socioeconomic status and the absence of intellectual stimulation (Gribbin, Schaie, & Parham, 1980), as well as having an inflexible personality

(Schaie, 1984) all increase the risk of cognitive decline in old age. This suggests that a significant component of the age-related declines in cognitive capacity are the result of "pathological" aging (i.e., they may be secondary to health or environmental insults), and are not representative of "normal" aging.

When social scientists define aging, they tend to focus primarily on role changes and social adjustment (see Rosow, 1985). Indeed, in her Presidential Address (to the American Sociological Association), Riley (1987) defined the social aging of individuals this way:

> As they age . . . they move through the stages of family life, school grades, career trajectories, into retirement and ultimate death. They are continually being reallocated to new sets of roles and resocialized to perform them. This movement with aging occurs partly by individual choice, but it is also channeled by the rules, linkages, and mechanisms governing role sequences within the social structure. (p. 4)

Thus, definitions of social aging are generally even more removed from chronological time than their biological or psychological counterparts. The reason for this is that the opportunity and timing of an individual's ascent into the next stage of the life course is subject to considerable external (and especially social) control.

Notice also the heavy emphasis here on the age-graded nature of the social structure (see Van Gennep, 1908; Linton, 1936; Parsons, 1951). At each age-grade individuals must learn the roles that they are expected to play that are associated with their current status. As they progress through the life course (i.e., as they pass from one age-grade to another), they are confronted with new statuses and their attendant roles to be mastered. According to Rosow (1985), it is only when they reach old age that individuals enter an age-grade of nonstatus that lacks well-defined and meaningful attendant roles. He argues that this accounts for the higher rates of depression and lower levels of self-esteem among the elderly.

An example of social aging involves the use of physician services by elderly Americans. In an examination of the Health Interview Survey data from 1972, 1976, and 1980, Wolinsky, Mosely, and Coe (1986) found that the use of physician services increased with age, but only until the birth cohorts under observation reached their eighth decade. At that point, their physician use began a steady and uninterrupted decline. This finding was unanticipated, inasmuch as all previous studies had detected continued age-related increases in physician use (see Haug, 1981; Wan, 1988).

It also posed a significant problem in interpretation given the absence of sociological explanations of why the elderly use more health services than the nonelderly in the first place (McKinlay, 1985). Indeed, sociologists who study health and health behavior have implicitly (if not explicitly) assumed (and demonstrated) that the need for health care, whether it be real or perceived, physiological or psychological, is the major reason for the use of health services (see Aday, Fleming, & Andersen, 1984; Wolinsky & Coe, 1984; Mechanic, 1988; Wolinsky et al., 1983). This need for health care was simply thought to increase as individuals aged, concomitant with natural (or perceived) processes of physiological deterioration. Therefore, it had been conventional sociological wisdom that as individuals aged, they used more health services.

That fundamentally biomedical explanation became much less plausible in the presence of data showing a decline in physician use concomitant with a continuing decline in health status. Borrowing on Brody's (1985) provocative work on intergenerational assistance and transfer, Wolinsky et al. suggested that the observed decline in physician use represented the substitution of informal services by the elders' children. They argue that this is plausible because (Wolinsky et al., 1986):

> a collection of related life-cycle changes—including the empty nest, reduced labor force participation, and other increases in pecuniary and nonpecuniary assets of the children of the oldest-old—enables their near-elderly children to increase significantly the informal supports and care that they can, and are called on to, provide for their parents. (p. 216)

Thus, changing social roles, in part brought about by the emergence of significant numbers of the oldest-old (see Rosenwaike, 1985) and their near-elderly children (see Torrey, 1985), appear to have altered the demand for physicians services among octogenarians.

Period Effects

It is not infrequent that the notion of history enters into discussions of aging and its role in the process of social change. Usually this involves some form of the admonition like "things were different back then," and that this accounts for changes in behavioral patterns. For example, consider the change in behavior before, during, and after King Arthur's legendary Camelot. For that matter, consider the fleeting hope and vitality that is sometimes described as the Camelot of the

Kennedy presidency (see Knoke & Hout, 1976). In these as well as other cases, a particular historical event had an impact on social change. Regardless of their nature, particular historical influences such as these are called period effects. The commonest characteristic of period effects is that they are external to the individual. Indeed, they represent changes in the environment in which the individual lives. These changes may occur at either the biological, psychological, or social level. Moreover, any given period effect might register an impact at two, or even at all three levels. It is also important to note that period effects do not necessarily affect all individuals, nor is the effect among affected individuals uniform. The reason for this is the differential opportunity for exposure to the period effect.

Consider, for example, the period effect on Americans of the Great Depression (see Elder, 1974, 1975; Elder & Liker, 1982). As a phenomenon, the Great Depression was external to any individual or group of individuals. It was also delimited to a particular place in historical time. Further, it had significant time-bound (i.e., temporary) effects at both the psychological level (such as increases in depression and suicide rates) and at the social level (such as the disruption and dislocation of family life, and the implementation of social welfare policies at the national level). These effects, however, did not impact on everyone (some industrial sectors and geographical locations were spared), nor did they affect all individuals equally (the working class, self-employed, and recent immigrants fared the worst). Thus, although the Great Depression produced a period effect, that effect is not uniform across all individuals.

At the biological level period effects frequently involve the alteration of the ecosystem. This may occur by accident, such as the recent case of the Soviet Union's Chernobyl nuclear reactor leakage, or by intent, such as the case of the fluoridation of water supplies in the United States since the 1960s. In both cases the outcome of the period effect is a shift (either upward or downward) in the disease burden. Beyond the effects of radiation poisoning, those who were exposed to the Chernobyl accident will likely develop higher incidence rates for most known cancers and other chronic disorders. Thus, their use of health services can be expected to increase. In contrast, Americans whose drinking water comes from fluoridated sources will likely have lower rates of dental caries than those whose water does not. That should result in fewer visits to the dentist (see Banting, 1984).

Period effects at the biological level, however, need not directly affect the ecosystem. Rather, they can provide individuals with a better defense system against environmentally based health threats.

Consider, for example, the impact of the introduction of polio vaccine in the mid-1950s. After a massive inoculation program, the threat of polio was eliminated worldwide (see Torrens, 1984). Twentieth-century medicine has provided many such period effects stemming from new discoveries and changes in treatment regimens.

An example of a period effect at the psychological level would be the increasing activism of lobbying groups for the elderly. Butler (1975) notes that the emergence of the "gray panther" movement and the rise of the American Association of Retired Persons (AARP) in the late 1960s and early 1970s had a considerable impact on changing the way the public, and the elderly themselves, viewed the aged. In addition to enhanced (but not yet important) social recognition by others, the elderly's self-esteem rose during this period (see also Achenbaum, 1985).

Binstock (1985), however, warns that this new-found political power of the elderly, whether it is real or only imagined, carries with it some rather negative consequences. As the budget deficit crisis intensified during the early 1980s, he argues that a distorted representation, such that the recently won services provided to the elderly are at the heart of the fiscal dilemma (i.e., "tabloid thinking"), might lead to a social and political backlash. The recent proposal by Callahan (1987) to eliminate a broad range of health services from the Medicare program for those older than 75 years of age suggests that Binstock may be right (see also Binstock & Kahana, 1988).

Three related period effects during the last five decades have dramatically altered the status of the elderly at the social level. Each one has involved deliberate actions on the part of the federal government. Moreover, they have all significantly affected the health and health behavior of elderly Americans. The three period effects are the implementation of the Social Security Program in the early 1930s, the introduction of Medicare and Medicaid in 1965, and the adoption of the prospective payment system with its diagnostic-related groups (DRGs) in 1983.

The enactment of the Social Security legislation was the harbinger of the American social welfare system (see Fischer, 1977). It provided a minimal subsistence income for eligible retiring workers. This at least partially mitigated the poverty that had typically been associated with retirement. In so doing it allowed an increased opportunity (at the discretion of its recipients) for health maintenance and the consumption of health services. More important, however, was its alteration of the social status of the elderly, resulting in the creation of an "entitlement mentality" (see Binstock, 1985).

Three decades later, the introduction of the Medicare and Medicaid Programs served to intensify this new social status for the elderly by specifically guaranteeing health care benefits (see Anderson, 1985). This substantially altered the health and health behavior of the elderly in two ways. First, on the demand side, it removed many of the socioeconomic barriers to the use of health services that had arisen concomitant with the rapidly rising cost of health care. Second, on the supply side, it provided considerable incentives (through guaranteed reimbursement on a fee-for-service basis) that motivated health care providers to seek out elderly patients (a group whom they would previously have avoided) for treatment. As a result, the elderly's consumption of health services increased dramatically.

With the shift in 1983 to DRGs (see Fetter, Shin, Freeman, Averill, & Thompson, 1980) as the reimbursement mechanism for Medicare, the incentive structure for health care providers was substantially altered. Under such an episode-based capitation system, the new incentives motivated health care providers to do less (i.e., to skimp) and to do even that less expensively (i.e., to substitute cheaper inputs) than before for any individual's particular episode of care, while at the same time to seek out more episodes (i.e., to generate more demand for their services). As a result, the number of hospital episodes involving elderly patients has increased at the same time that the average length of stay and associated costs have decreased (see Wolinsky, 1988).

Cohort Effects

Just as the notion of particular historical periods enters into the discussion of the aging process, so too does the concept of particular cohorts of individuals. Cohorts were explicitly brought to the attention of social scientists as a critical element in the study of social change by Ryder in 1965. He argued that much (but not all) of the process of social change could be explained by "demographic metabolism," or the structural transformation that occurs when new birth cohorts replace their predecessors in the age-graded status hierarchy. In the aggregate, this is how society counterbalances the aging and the ultimate death of its members.

The utility of studying cohorts, as opposed to merely studying age-groups or periods, stems from their definition. Cohorts are typically delimited as including all those individuals born during a given interval, such as between 1900 and 1910, although this is not necessarily the case (see Schaie & Hertzog [1985] who have begun to argue for the construction of "nonchronological" cohorts based on the point in an individual's life at which an index event of interest occurs [like the death of a spouse]). As such, the members of a given birth cohort age and experience the same historical events at the same time.

This point has important implications for the analysis of social change. Ryder (1965) notes:

> Each new cohort makes fresh contact with the contemporary social heritage and carries the impress of the encounter through life. This confrontation has been called the intersection of the innovative and the conservative forces in history. . . . The members of any cohort are entitled to participate in only one slice of life—their unique location in the stream of history. Because it embodies a temporally specific version of the heritage, each cohort is differentiated from all others, despite the minimization of variability by symbolically perpetuated institutions and by hierarchically graduated structures of authority. (p. 844)

Thus, one would expect that a particular cohort's brush with a historical event at its unique stage (i.e., age-grade) in the life cycle might result in the development and maintenance of an enduring and distinctive behavioral response or personality trait.

Elder (1974, 1975) has documented just such an effect related to the Great Depression. He focuses on those born around the turn of the century, who would have been in their late 20s and early 30s during the economic collapse of the 1930s. The reason that this particular birth cohort would be most likely to be adversely affected by the Great Depression is that they were losing their jobs, their economic security, and their sense of meaning in life precisely at a point in the life cycle when such things traditionally did not occur. Having incurred such losses when they were most unexpected, the members of this cohort became far more self-reliant and frugal than the members of other cohorts. In a sense, the members of this cohort became far more sensitive to the potential for economic hardship and the need to be prepared for it.

Subsequent research has underscored just how enduring this cohort effect has been. Using longitudinal data on the women in this birth cohort, Elder and Liker (1982) have shown that the earlier economic hardships had a considerable effect on the women's health and well-being 40 years later. For working class women (who faced the greatest and most permanent economic hardships) the results were particularly adverse, whereas for middle-class women (who faced less severe and more temporary economic setbacks) the effect was relatively benign. On the one hand, these data demonstrate that the effects of being in a particular birth cohort are not necessarily felt by all of its members (see also Maddox, 1979; Palmore, 1978; Riley, 1973; Rosow, 1978). Conversely, these data provide clear evidence that cohort effects can be quite enduring.

Cohort effects can also result from technological developments. Glenn (1976) describes, for example, the impact of the availability of reliable birth control devices beginning in the 1960s:

> the cohort of females now in young adulthood differs markedly from cohorts only a few years older in capability for voluntary fertility control; its members are the first females able to plan and begin a career with high assurance that it will not be interrupted involuntarily by pregnancy. (p. 902)

This has remarkable implications for the ability of this cohort to alter its life-course development from traditional patterns. Indeed, its fertility rates are substantially lower and its age at first birth is substantially higher than those that came before it. This has had important effects on the opportunity structure of the cohort that followed because of its reduced size (see Hogan, 1981).

Although the preceding examples have focused on cohort effects of a fundamentally social and psychological nature, they can also be of a more strictly biological nature. One need only consider the case of thalidomide and diethylstilbestrol (DES) babies to make the point. At the time that the physicians of mothers of this rather select cohort recommended the ingestion of these drugs, they were considered to be the best (and presumed safest, albeit experimental) regimens available for the treatment of morning sickness and the inability to carry the pregnancy to term. Aside from the congenital abnormalities of the thalidomide babies and the higher risk for ovarian and uterine cancer among the DES babies, it is not yet known what other problems and maladies will emerge as this unique cohort ages.

More broadly evident cohort effects on the health and health behavior of the elderly can be discussed by referring back to the Great Depression example. Building on the work of Elder (1974, 1975) and Butler (1975), Wolinsky et al. (1986) contrasted those older cohorts who lived through the turbulent 1930s as young or middle-aged adults with those subsequent cohorts who were of comparable age and life cycle position during World War II or later. On the one hand, these authors hypothesized that the older cohorts might use fewer health services in the 1980s because of their aversion to accepting or relying on external supports, such as Medicare and Medicaid (which are common sources of payment for health care services among the elderly). Conversely, Wolinsky et al. (1986) expected the younger cohorts to use more health services because they had, since their formative years, been socialized to the "entitlement mentality" that began with Social Security, was augmented by the G.I. Bill of Rights, and solidified under Medicare and Medicaid (see also Binstock, 1985). Unfortunately, the issue is not fully resolved. Although the preliminary data that they present on the per capita number of physician visits is consistent with their expectations, the data on hospital use is not.

Putting the Pieces Together

The preceding sections indicate that good reasons exist to anticipate age, period, and cohort effects at the biological, psychological, and social levels. That much is relatively straightforward. What is less obvious, however, is the conceptual framework that accommodates the systematic integration and articulation of these effects. The rudiments of such an approach began to occur in 1965. In that year, not only did Ryder publish his pivotal exegesis of the role of cohorts in the process of social change (discussed earlier), but Schaie published a landmark paper presenting a general model for the analysis of developmental processes.

As indicated earlier, Schaie (1965) was involved in the debate about the question of whether age-related changes in intelligence and cognition existed. Up to that time, most research attempting to address this question was of a cross-sectional nature. In those studies, a significant negative correlation was found between age and intelligence (as measured by various standardized tests). Based on that evidence, most researchers argued that intelligence and cognition systematically and inevitably declined with age.

Schaie (1965), however, thought that although one could construct a good theoretical argument for an aging effect, one could construct an equally good (and he believed better) theoretical argument for a cohort effect. In this case, he hypothesized that the marked and continual gains in educational attainment benefiting each successive birth cohort might account for the aging effect being found in these cross-sectional studies. Moreover, he noted that the effects of age and period could not be separated in data from a single cross-sectional survey.

Figure 1.1 can be used to demonstrate Schaie's (1965) point. Along one axis is the date at which any given measurement of the

Date of measurement

Date of birth	1860	1880	1900	1920	1940	1960	1980	2000	2020	2040	2060
1860	0	20	40	60	80	100	—	—	—	—	—
1880	—	0	20	40	60	80	100	—	—	—	—
1900	—	—	0	20	40	60	80	100	—	—	—
1920	—	—	—	0	20	40	60	80	100	—	—
1940	—	—	—	—	0	20	40	60	80	100	—
1960	—	—	—	—	—	0	20	40	60	80	100

Figure 1.1 Schale's (1965) Illustration of the Relationship Between Age, Time of Measurement, and Date of Birth.

Source: Adapted from Schaie, K.W. (1965). A general model for the study of developmental problems. *Psychological Bulletin* 64:92-107, © 1965 by the American Psychological Association. Adapted by permission.

respondents' intelligence might have been taken, using 20-year intervals. The other axis indicates the date of birth for any cohort that might be constructed, also using 20-year intervals. The numbers in each of the cells indicate the age of that particular birth cohort (i.e., row) during that particular round of measurement (i.e., column).

Looking only at the data that would be obtained from one particular cross-sectional survey in Figure 1.1, say that conducted in 1960, brings the problem into full relief. Although the entire range of adult age-groups would be represented (i.e., the 2nd, 4th, 6th, 8th, and 10th decades), each of those age-groups is fully populated by members of a unique birth cohort (i.e., each was born at a different point in history). Thus, by just having that one column's worth of data, it would be impossible to separate out the effects of age from those of cohort. That is, how would one know if the age-group differences in intelligence observed in that cross-sectional study were due to the developmental decay of cognitive functioning, or to the differential educational attainment of successive birth cohorts?

This might have lead some researchers to argue that the field should shift to longitudinal studies. In such studies measurements on individuals from one or more birth cohorts are taken at one point in time (e.g., 1920), and are then repeated on these same individuals at subsequent points in time. Schaie (1965), however, was quick to point out the problems with that approach as well. Assuming (for simplicity) that only one birth cohort was to be followed longitudinally, such a design would be equivalent to the data stream represented in any given row of Figure 1.1. For example, if the 1860 birth cohort had its intelligence measured every 20 years until its members reached age 100, the design would be that of the first row. Although this would have solved the cohort problem that plagues cross-sectional studies, it introduces another. Moving from left to right within the first row would indicate not only aging effects but also period effects. The reason is that although the 1860 birth cohort ages 20 years as it moves from column to column, it also ages through different periods of history. Thus, longitudinal designs also fail to provide measures of "pure" aging effects.

At about the same time that Schaie (1965) was working on the methodological issues of obtaining aging effects net of those of period or cohort, Riley, Foner, Moore, Hess, and Roth (1968) were asked by the Russell Sage Foundation to summarize what was known about social studies of the aging process (see Riley, 1987). They, however, took a more conceptual approach that eventually resulted in the formalization of the age-stratification perspective (see Riley, 1972,

1976, 1985; Riley, Foner, & Waring, 1988; Riley, Johnson, & Foner, 1972).

Riley's (1972) original notion of the age-stratification perspective is graphically portrayed in Figure 1.2 (see Riley, Foner, & Waring, 1988). Notice that although the format is somewhat different than that of Figure 1.1, the logic is similar. In Figure 1.2 each diagonal bar (labelled A, B, or C) represents the life course of a particular cohort that ages biologically, psychologically, and socially as discussed earlier. The fact that there are several diagonal bars represents the continuing entrance of new birth cohorts into society. The vertical bars indicate that at any particular point in time, a single cross-sectional survey captures people in different age-strata, reflecting the age-graded role structure of society. Finally, the horizontal axis indicates that society itself may or may not change over historical time. When taken together, these factors illustrate the "dynamic interplay" between the two processes of individual aging and social change.

It is the notion of such a "dynamic interplay" that represents the major contribution of the age-stratification approach, because both aging and social change had long been topics *separately* addressed by social scientists (see Riley, 1987). The iterative articulation of aging and

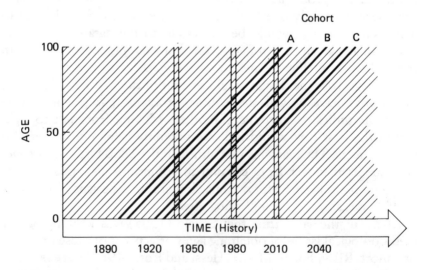

Figure 1.2 Riley's (1972) illustration of the age stratification system.

Source: Riley, M. W., Foner, A., & Waring. J. Sociology of age. In Neil J. Smelser, ed., *Handbook of Sociology*, p. 245, © 1988 by Sage Publications. Reprinted by permission of Sage Publications, Inc.

social change is built on three general principles, the first of which focuses on cohort differences in aging. Riley (1987) explains this principle by referring to Figure 1.2:

> it is the whole succession of diagonal bars—the flow of cohorts—that draws attention to the significant fact here: because each cohort is born at a particular date, it lives through a unique segment of historical time and confronts its own particular sequence of social and environmental events and changes. Thus it is cohort comparison that brings us inexorably to the first principle (early formulated by Ryder [1965]), namely: because society changes, people in different cohorts age in different ways. (p. 4)

Riley uses the retirement of American men to illustrate this principle, noting the difference in expectations about how many years would be spent in retirement between cohorts born early in this century and those born later.

The second (and logically related) principle focuses on cohort influence on social change, which Riley (1987) explains this way:

> because members of successive cohorts age in new ways, they contribute to changes in the social structure. . . . As society moves through time, the age strata of people and roles are altered. The people in particular age strata are no longer the same people; they have been replaced by younger entrants from more recent cohorts, with more recent life experiences. (p. 4)

Using the retirement example once again, Riley illustrates this principle by focusing on the social change brought about by the increasing ratio (i.e., tax burden) of beneficiaries of to contributors to Social Security.

The dynamic interplay between these first two principles is illustrated as follows (Riley, 1987):

> In response to social change, millions of individuals in a cohort begin to develop new age-typical patterns and regularities of behavior (changes in aging); these behavior patterns then become defined as age-appropriate norms and rules, are reinforced by "authorities," and thereby become institutionalized in the structure of society (social change); in turn, these changes in age norms and social structures redirect age-related behaviors (further changes in aging). (p. 4)

It is through this dialectic between aging and social change that alterations are made in both the aging process and the social structure.

What is perhaps even more important, however, is the third principle. It involves the asynchrony between the occurrence of the micro (i.e., aging) and macro (i.e., social change) forces. Riley (1987) explains this as follows:

> Each dynamism has it own tempo. Within each cohort, people moving along the axis of the life course are born and die according to a rhythm set by the approximate current length of the human lifetime. In contrast, social change moves . . . along its own axis of historical time; it is influenced by imbalances, strains, and conflicts within the age stratification system, as well as by external social and environmental events or evolutionary changes in the organism. (p. 5)

Thus, although a birth cohort is socialized to the full range of age-graded norms when it is young (such as how much education is necessary to get ahead, or what it is like to be old), social change frequently makes those expectations obsolete by the time the cohort reaches the respective age-grades. The likelihood of asynchrony is especially great whenever technological change is rapid (e.g., the remarkable asynchrony brought about by the computer revolution).

Failure to recognize the implications of these three principles may (and frequently has) lead to four general misinterpretations (see Riley, 1973, 1981). The first is the life-course fallacy, in which the differences between age-groups found in cross-sectional data are taken as indicators of aging effects, which they are not. Rather, these differences are the tools to be used in examining age-strata effects. Cohort-centrism is the second fallacy. It involves the erroneous assumption that the members of all other cohorts will age in the same way that the particular cohort under study has aged. Age-reification is the third fallacy. Here, chronological age is mistakenly understood as having a causal effect in and of itself. Similarly, the fourth fallacy is reifying historical time. This involves treating period effects as causal without specifying why they might be important in making sense out of particular shifts in the aging process. Riley notes that although much of the earlier literature was understandably plagued by these misinterpretations (see Riley et al., 1968), some researchers regrettably continue to make the same mistakes (Riley, 1985, 1987).

STANDARD COHORT ANALYTIC TECHNIQUES

Perhaps the most salient contribution of the age-stratification perspective is its emphasis on the importance of considering all three (i.e., age, period, and cohort) effects when approaching any given substantive issue. The reason for this is that to consider any one of the effects without regard for the other two is to arrive, except in extremely rare "pure" cases (to be illustrated later), at a misleading diagnostic assessment. For example, consider the case of attempting to assess only one of these effects, say aging, on the percentage of persons who see a dentist at least once during a given calendar year. Sound a priori reasons exist to assume that aging effects would be present. From a developmental standpoint, one would expect the progression of dental disease to result in more frequent visits for restorative and replacement purposes. Thus, one would likley hypothesize a direct relationship between age and dental contact, assuming some adjustment for edentulism. That much seems intuitively straightforward (see Beck, 1984; Conrad, 1982; Evashwick, Conrad, & Lee, 1982; Kiyak, 1984).

To stop there, however, would be too great of an oversimplification. For if one assumes that oral health behavior is a relatively stable lifelong trait secured by early adulthood, then one would also expect to find cohort differences reflecting any changes occurring in normative behavioral expectations between successive birth cohorts' formative years. Given that expectations for personal oral hygiene have increased dramatically during this century, one would likely hypothesize that significant cohort succession effects would gradually increase aggregate dental contact rates (see Kiyak, 1987; Wolinksy & Arnold, 1989). The historical introduction of water and toothpaste fluoridation, as well as the increasing reliance on dental hygienists and assistants would also lead one to expect period effects in dental contact rates (see Department of Health and Human Services, 1982). On the one hand, the resulting decline in dental caries would likely lead to a reduction in contact rates (see Banting, 1984). Conversely, the increase in access to dental services brought about by the introduction of auxiliary dental personnel would likely lead to an increase in use (see Wolinsky, 1988). Thus, failure to simultaneously consider period and cohort effects in an assessment of the relationship between aging and dental contact rates would likely yield erroneous results.

Logic of Cohort Methods

A logical outgrowth of the age-stratification perspective has been the development of a general class of methods that permit one to begin simultaneously assessing age, period, and cohort effects. These methods are generally classified under the rubric "cohort methods" (see Glenn, 1977; Mason & Fienberg, 1984). They may be further classified into two subtypes: panel studies (sometimes referred to as "longitudinal" studies), and sequential cross-sectional studies (sometimes referred to as "synthetic" studies). Both involve tracking two or more birth cohorts during two or more periods. The fundamental difference between them is that panel studies (such as the Framingham Heart Study, or the Longitudinal Retirement History Study) follow the same individuals over time, whereas sequential cross-sectional studies (such as can be constructed by using the annual cross-sectional surveys of the General Social Survey, or the Health Interview Survey [HIS] track different representative samples of the various birth cohorts over time. As a result, intraindividual change can only be assessed in panel studies. Sequential cross-sectional studies are restricted to assessments of interindividual (or more aggregate-level) change.

Although the panel type of cohort studies have obvious advantages, they are not without their own disadvantages (see Maddox & Campbell, 1985). Principal among these are the opportunity costs of identifying and obtaining baseline data on an appropriate set of birth cohorts, and then continuing to track those same individuals over the next several decades to obtain subsequent waves of follow-up data. Among these opportunity costs are the logistical problems of tracking the cohorts' members, the ambiguities of procuring funding support over such a prolonged period, and the dedication and patience of the investigators to remain committed to such a long-term project. Although recent commitments from the National Institute on Aging to support "The Establishment of Populations for Epidemiologic Studies of the Elderly" (EPESE; see Cornoni-Huntley, Ostfeld, Taylor, & Wallace, 1986) are an important step forward in securing such data for eventual public use, limitations in sample size, geographical representation, and the projected number and timing of follow-ups will limit their potential as a panacea.

Because of these opportunity costs, most cohort studies have involved the use of sequential cross-sectional analysis. Such analysis is based on the construction of standard cohort tables like the one shown in Table 1.1, which has clear and logical ties to Figures 1.1 and 1.2. The issue under examination in this table is the percentage of Americans who reported a "great deal" of interest in politics. The table itself consists of data (the percentage so interested) taken from three cross-sectional surveys (i.e., 1952, 1960, and 1968) for each of the seven birth cohorts identified (i.e., those aged 21 to 28 in 1952, those aged 29 to 36 in 1952, up to those aged 69 to 76 in 1952). This illustrates an important technical requirement for the construction of

Table 1.1 Percentage of Respondents to Gallup Public Opinion Polls Who Reported a "GreatDeal" of Interest in Politics in the United States During 1952, 1960, and 1968, by Age-Group

	Survey year		
Age-group	1952	1960	1968
21-28	19.0	18.4	18.7
29-36	22.0	22.3	17.4
37-44	24.1	24.8	17.0
45-52	28.6	21.7	20.5
53-60	30.7	28.7	19.0
61-68	33.8	27.8	18.9
69-76	37.3	30.0	23.0
Grand mean	25.7	24.2	18.9

Source: Adapted from Glenn, N.D. *Cohort Analysis*, p. 11, © 1977 by Sage Publications. Reprinted by permission of Sage Publications, Inc.

standard cohort tables. The intervals between the points in time (i.e., the surveys that identify the columns) must correspond in years to the intervals that are used to delineate the birth cohorts (i.e., the width of the designated age-groups that identify the rows).

When such a standard cohort table has been constructed, the identification of age, period, and cohort effects would appear to become rather straightforward. Age effects may be determined by examining *intra*cohort differences (i.e., by reading diagonally down and to the right). This allows one to compare, for example, the reported level of interest in politics from a representative sample of the cohort aged 21 to 28 in 1952 (which was 19.0%) with that reported by a different representative sample of that same cohort 8 years later (in 1960) when its members were then aged 29 to 36 (which was 22.3%), and to compare them both with that reported by a yet different representative sample of that same cohort 8 years later (in 1968) when its members were then aged 37 to 44 (which was 17.0%). One could then repeat this process for the six remaining birth cohorts, presumably paying particular attention to those aging effects that were consistently replicated across the different birth cohorts.

Period effects may be determined by comparing the same age-group at one point in time with that in another point in time (i.e., by reading across the rows). This allows one to compare, for example, the reported level of interest in politics of a representative sample of those aged 21 to 28 in 1952 (which was, again, 19.0%) with that reported by a representative sample of those aged 21 to 28 in 1960 (which was 18.4%), and to compare them both with that reported by a representative sample of those aged 21 to 28 in 1968 (which was 18.7%). Here again, one would presumably pay greater attention to those period effects that were consistently replicated across all age-groups.

Finally, cohort membership effects may be determined by examining *inter*cohort changes (i.e., by reading down the columns). This allows one to compare, for example, the reported level of interest in politics of a representative sample of those aged 21 to 28 in 1952 (which was, once again, 19.0%) with that reported by representative samples of those aged 29 to 36, 37 to 44, 45 to 52, 53 to 60, 61 to 68, and 69 to 76 in 1952 (which were, respectively, 22.0%, 24.1%, 28.6%, 30.7%, 33.8%, and 37.3%). Once again, one would presumably pay greater attention to those cohort effects that were consistently replicated across all periods.

Three Obstacles to Interpretation

The interpretation of age, period, and cohort effects in standard cohort tables, however, is not quite so straightforward. Three general problems may complicate matters: sampling error, compositional change, and statistical confounding (see Glenn, 1977). It is important to note here that these problems exist regardless of whether the study design employs a panel or a sequential cross-sectional approach. Indeed, the only difference between the two approaches lies in the methods that are used to resolve the problems.

Sampling error problems in cohort analyses are no different from those faced when using other methodological techniques. Whenever samples of a population are used, the resulting point estimates (such as the percentages shown in the cells of Table 1.1) are subject to sampling error. That is to say that there are implicit confidence intervals around each percentage reported in the table. The magnitude of the confidence intervals depends on the heterogeneity of the target behavior within each cell (typically measured by the standard deviation) as well as the sample size within each cell. As the heterogeneity declines or as the sample size increases, the confidence interval shrinks.

The sampling error problem, therefore, can be minimized when large-scale surveys are available. Moreover, as with other statistical techniques, inferential tests can be applied. Although these are not yet well developed specifically for cohort analysis (Glenn, 1977), the general logic is to ensure that the criteria for statistical significance require the magnitude of any observed effects to exceed that expected simply because a sample was taken. Interpreted conservatively, this would mean that for any two cells under comparison in Table 1.1 to be considered as having different levels of interest in politics, the confidence intervals of the two point estimates (percentages) could not overlap. A more liberal test would require only that each of the two point estimates (percentages) fall outside of the 95% confidence interval of the other (see Wolinsky & Arnold, 1989; Wolinsky, Arnold, & Nallapati, 1988).

Compositional change refers to the problem that as cohorts age, they suffer attrition from the death of some of their members. This is especially problematic when cohort techniques are applied to data on elderly adults inasmuch as they have higher mortality rates. If the survivors differ from the decedents on any key characteristics under study, then the interpretation of age, period, or cohort effects becomes obfuscated in much the same way that experimental mortality plagues the internal validity of randomized trials (see Schaie & Hertzog, 1985). The reason is that as the amount of compositional change increases, it becomes progressively more difficult to partition accurately any observed change between "true" changes (i.e., those related to age, period, and cohort effects) and those brought about by mortality induced attrition.

Two general means exist for dealing with the threats to internal validity that are introduced by compositional change. In panel studies it is often possible to analyze the survivors separately from the decedents (see Mossey & Shapiro, 1985; Mossey, Havens, & Wolinsky, 1988). Any differences in the parameter estimates between the separate assessments can then be credited to compositional change. Because different representative samples of cohorts are studied in sequential cross-sectional designs, a different approach must be used. Here, various standardization or adjustment procedures can be introduced to compensate for any changes in the distributions of key characteristics of the cohorts over time (see Glenn, 1977). This approach is restricted by the availability of such adjusting or standardizing factors in the data.

Despite the difficulties introduced by the sampling error and compositional change issues, it is the statistical confounding that is most problematical for cohort analysis. The statistical confounding results from the fact that there is a linear dependency in which the basic effects of two factors (i.e., age, period, and cohort) are both involved in each diagonal, row, or column comparison (see Glenn, 1977; also note that the statistical confounding issue is frequently referred to as the identification problem, the technical resolution of which [or attempts thereof] will be addressed in detail later in this chapter). For example, age and cohort effects are both represented in column comparisons, because the cohorts to be compared have attained different ages. Similarly, cohort and period effects are both evidenced in row comparisons, because different birth cohorts are being compared at different points in history. Age and period effects are both involved in diagonal comparisons, because the cohorts not only age, they age into new historical periods. Thus, the separation of age, period, and cohort effects by visual inspection of standard cohort tables is difficult unless the observed effects are both pronounced and consistent across all comparisons, which is a rather rare occurrence.

Visual Inspection of Standard Cohort Tables

Tables 1.2 to 1.4 help illustrate the method of visually inspecting standard cohort tables. All three tables contain hypothetical data concerning the percentage of persons in their 40s, 50s, 60s, 70s, and 80s who have seen a dentist during 1960, 1970, and 1980. Thus, the number of years between surveys matches exactly the width of the age-group used to identify the cohorts, satisfying the technical requirement for standard cohort table construction. To simplify matters, each table displays "pure" (i.e., unadulterated) effects related solely to age, period, or cohort based on the expectations described earlier.

An examination of Table 1.2 reveals only aging effects. As each cohort ages 10 years and their teeth naturally deteriorate, the dental contact rate increases 10 percentage points. The one exception is that dental contact rates level off when each cohort reaches their eighth decade, reflecting the (arbitrarily chosen) effects of the onset of edentulism. Note that no period effects exist. This is evidenced by the equality of the percentages within the rows. Similarly, the pattern of variation between the age-groups within each column is identical across the columns. Thus, no cohort effects exist. Indeed, the only

Table 1.2 Standard Cohort Table Illustrating "Pure" Age Effects Using Hypothetical Data on Percentage of Respondents Having Seen a Dentist During 12 Months Preceding the Interview

	Survey year		
Age-group	1960	1970	1980
40-49	50	50	50
50-59	60	60	60
60-69	70	70	70
70-79	80	80	80
80-89	80	80	80
Grand mean	68	68	68

effect occurring in this table is an aging one. That explains why the grand mean remains the same for all 3 years.

Table 1.3, in contrast, contains only period effects. Here, the increase over time of water and toothpaste fluoridation has resulted in a 10-percentage-point decline every 10 years. This decline is the same within all row comparisons. It is important to note that in this table no variation exists between the age-groups during any particular year. That explains why from year to year the grand mean declines the same amount (10 percentage points) as the change for each age-group. Thus, period effects are analogous to shift parameters in which the distribution by age-group within a given year is multiplied by a constant to produce the distribution for a subsequent year.

Pure cohort effects are shown in Table 1.4. Here the pattern is that of cohort succession, in which each new cohort enters the table with a dental contact rate 10 percentage points higher than its predecessor. Note that no aging effects exist. That is, the dental contact rate of each cohort remains the same regardless of how much it ages. Also note that the changes observed across the rows are in the opposite direction of those observed down the columns. As a result of the cohort effect shown here, the increases in the grand means are identical to those between successive cohorts.

Table 1.3 Standard Cohort Table Illustrating "Pure" Period Effects Using Hypothetical Data on Percentage of Respondents Having Seen a Dentist During 12 Months Preceding the Interview

	Survey year		
Age-group	1960	1970	1980
40-49	60	50	40
50-59	60	50	40
60-69	60	50	40
70-79	60	50	40
80-89	60	50	40
Grand mean	60	50	40

The interpretation of standard cohort tables with "real" data, however, is seldom so straightforward. Two major reasons exist for this difficulty. First, it is infrequent that a single, "pure" effect can be found. Indeed, each of the preceding dental contact rate illustrations is based on sound a priori theory. Therefore, one would expect to find some amount of age, *and* period, *and* cohort effects. That introduces considerable complexity. Second, with the exception of the adjustment for edentulism among those in their eighth decade in Table 1.2, all three examples represent only additive effects. That is, the aging effect was the same for all cohorts and during all periods; the cohort effect was the same for all age-groups and during all periods; and the period effect was the same for all age-groups and all cohorts.

Those are not altogether reasonable assumptions, however. For example, the period (i.e., fluoridation) effects would likely be greater for younger cohorts than for older cohorts, because much dental disease is of a progressive and developmental nature (this would be an example of a period-cohort interaction). Similarly, the aging (i.e., deterioration) effects would likely be smaller for younger cohorts because of their greater exposure to fluoridation during their formative years (this would be an example of an age-period interaction). The cohort (i.e., differential normative expectations) effects would likely be larger in more recent periods when personal oral hygiene became more fashionable (this would be an example of a cohort-period interaction).

A return to Table 1.1 provides an opportunity to inspect visually what appears at first glance to be a deceivingly simple standard cohort table. Again, the dependent variable of interest in this table is the percentage of Americans who reported a "great deal" of interest in politics to Gallup pollsters in 1952, 1960, and 1968. Applying the methods illustrated earlier reveals two important if not trying points. First, no "pure" effects exist. Rather, a little bit of everything appears to be happening. Second, what is happening is not occurring consistently across all diagonal, row, or column comparisons. This indicates the presence of statistical interaction between age, period, and cohort.

Some important patterns (or subpatterns) of effects are in Table 1.1, however. At the most general level, a cohort effect appears to exist (albeit an impure one) such that older cohorts who express a greater interest in politics are being replaced by younger cohorts who are less interested in politics. A relatively consistent aging effect also appears to exist such that as cohorts age, their interest in politics declines somewhat. These effects are joined by an apparent age-period interaction effect reflecting an upward shift in interest in politics during 1960, but only for the two youngest age-groups. Similarly, there appears to be an age-period interaction effect reflecting an accelera-

Table 1.4 Standard Cohort Table Illustrating "Pure" Cohort Effects Using Hypothetical Data on Percentage of Respondents Having Seen a Dentist During 12 Months Preceding the Interview

Age-group	Survey year		
	1960	1970	1980
40-40	60	70	80
50-59	50	60	70
60-69	40	50	60
70-79	30	40	50
80-89	20	30	40
Grand mean	40	50	60

tion of the decline in interest in politics during the late 1960s, but
only for those over 60 years of age. Finally, an anomaly seems to exist
in that the interest in politics among the youngest age-group remains
stable across all the periods.

This is not as straightforward an interpretation as that given to
Tables 1.2 to 1.4. Nonetheless, ad hoc explanations (which could
have been hypothesized a priori) can be fitted to those patterns. It can
be argued that the general interest in politics among younger cohorts
is less than that among their older counterparts because of the latter
having lived through the Great Depression, and the remarkable political and social reforms that emerged from it (see Elder, 1974, 1975).
In essence, this view holds that because the economic and social
environments have improved so much and been so relatively stable
during the formative years of members of the younger cohorts, they
are less motivated to be politically active. The age-related decline in
being interested in politics can be argued as consistent with many
developmental theories (see Knoke & Hout, 1976). They suggest that
as adults mature, their interests shift from external factors (like politics) to more personal concerns (such as career development and
recreational activities).

The three other patterns require more effort at explanation, inasmuch as they represent the interaction of two main effects. One can
account for them, however. The first age-period interaction probably
reflects the special appeal of one of the 1960 presidential candidates,
John F. Kennedy, to younger voters. His candidacy may have been
sufficiently attractive to the two youngest cohorts to overcompensate
effectively for the traditionally anticipated decline in their interest
in politics, but only for that one point in time (see White, 1961).
The second age-period interaction probably reflects the extra decline
in politics among the elderly brought about by the establishment of
Medicare and Medicaid in 1965. Having achieved such important
entitlements, the elderly may have turned their attention to other
more personal concerns (see Knoke & Hout 1976). Finally, the
apparent anomaly of the stability of the youngest age-group's interest in politics over time may reflect the fact that the first time
one becomes eligible to vote is such a novel experience that it results
in an unusually keen interest in the political process (see Pomper,
1976).

Regardless of the validity of the preceding ad hoc interpretations,
two important points must be made from the visual inspection of
Table 1.1. The first is that *the cohort analyst relies on theoretical* (and
not statistical) *grounds to explain the general* (i.e., the additive or main)

effects of age, period, or cohort. The importance of identifying those theoretical grounds (which may consist of prior knowledge or explicit assumptions; see Cohn, 1972) before the visual inspection of the tables cannot be emphasized enough. Although this a priori reliance on theory is no different than that involved in any form of analysis (see Knoke & Hout, 1976; Mason & Fienberg, 1984; Mason, Mason, Winsborough, & Poole, 1976), the remarkable complexity of cohort analysis simply makes it all the more important (see Glenn, 1976, 1977, 1989; McRae & Brody, 1989; Schaie & Hertzog, 1985). Thus, the first rule of thumb in cohort analysis is to state one's theoretical expectations explicitly for the main effects up-front.

The second important point to emerge from the visual inspection of Table 1.1 involves the interaction effects. Although interaction effects may be anticipated before the analysis (in which case the a priori reasons for them should be explicitly stated up-front, just as one does for the main effects), most interaction effects will likely be discovered serendipitously. Explaining such effects requires a significant reliance on understanding the historical context in which they occur (such information can be thought of as a "side-bar" to the data actually presented in the standard cohort table [see Glenn, 1976, 1977; Palmore, 1978]). Although this is fundamentally no different than the logic used to interpret interaction effects that are estimated in other forms of analysis (such as multiple regression; see Lewis-Beck, 1980), the problem is intensified in cohort analysis because the visual inspection of the tables involves the assessment of all possible interaction terms. This problem increases the likelihood of identifying false-positive (i.e., Type II) interaction effects in cohort analysis. Thus, the second rule of thumb in cohort analysis is to *be skeptical in accepting the interpretation of an interaction effect,* especially if it involves only an isolated occurrence or two.

Glenn (1977) has gone beyond these two general rules to suggest four more practical guidelines that should govern the confidence expressed in any particular cohort analysis. The conditions under which Glenn (1977) believes identified patterns should be given credence include:

(1) patterns predicted by hypotheses well-grounded in theory, (2) monotonic, or almost monotonic, variation in a row, column, or cohort diagonal, (3) patterns common to several rows, columns, or cohort diagonals, and (4) patterns similar to those shown by other cohort studies with the same or similar dependent variables. (pp. 41–42)

These guidelines serve as a more concrete operationalization of the two rules of thumb presented earlier. Both emphasize that cohort analysis should be firmly rooted in theory, and that more consistently observed patterns should carry the greatest weight.

Statistical Resolution of Identification Problem

As indicated earlier, the greatest obstacle to the interpretation of standard cohort tables is the identification or statistical confounding problem (i.e., when the two dimensions of the standard cohort table are used to isolate the three effects of age, period, and cohort). Although it is generally recognized that the resolution of this issue ultimately rests on one's theory (either in terms of knowing or assuming that one of the effects is equal to zero; see Cohn, 1972); much work has been done during the past two decades to develop statistical techniques to assist cohort analysts in their deliberations. In particular, Mason and colleagues (see Mason, Mason, Winsborough, & Poole, 1973; Fienberg & Mason, 1978; Mason & Fienberg, 1984; Smith, Mason, & Fienberg, 1982) have presented what has come to be referred to as the "accounting formula" (or "framework" or "specification"). Despite, or perhaps because of, the considerable controversy surrounding this approach (see Glenn, 1976, 1977; Knoke & Hout, 1976; Mason et al., 1976; Palmore, 1978; Rodgers, 1982a, 1982b; Smith et al., 1982), it warrants further elaboration here.

To grasp the identification problem intuitively, consider again the model presented in Schaie's (1965) classic discussion of the problems in studying developmental issues. Figure 1.1 illustrates these problems well. Note two related points here. First, many empty cells exist, which results from the fact that these birth cohorts only lived through certain periods at certain ages. Thus, there are no observations of the 1860 birth cohort in 1980, nor are there any observations of the 1960 birth cohort in 1940. As a result, it is impossible to say with any certainty how similar or different any two cohorts would have behaved had they been of the same age at the same point.

It is the second point, however, that lies at the heart of the identification problem. Figure 1.1 demonstrates that if the year in which the data were collected (i.e., the period) and the year in which the cohort were born (i.e., the cohort) are both known, then the age of that cohort at that point in time is unequivocally fixed. Equation 1.1 expresses this in mathematical notation:

$$A = P - C \tag{1.1}$$

and can be demonstrated by using the example of determining the age of the 1860 birth cohort (C) when measured during 1940 (P). As Equation 1.2 indicates, the arithmetic is straightforward:

$$A = 1940 - 1860 = 80 \qquad (1.2)$$

Moreover, the same identification problem holds for any of the three effects (i.e., age, period, or cohort) when the other two are known.

The reader familiar with the use of dummy variables in multiple regression analysis (see Polissar & Diehr, 1982) will see that this is same kind of problem that occurs there. That is, if the parent variable, say religious preference, has four categories (e.g., Protestant, Catholic, Jew, and other), then only three dummy variables can be included in the model. The value of the fourth dummy variable would be un-equivocally determined by those of the other three. The three esti-mated coefficients measure the difference between the religious pref-erence of the group they represent and that of the group whose dummy variable was omitted (which is traditionally called the refer-ence category).

Schaie (1965), and subsequently Baltes (1968), tried to resolve the identification problem statistically by the application of analysis of variance techniques. The use of such a two-factor framework on a three-factor problem, however, could not succeed. In contrast, the accounting formula of Mason et al. (1973) essentially employs a multiple classification analysis framework that builds on Cohn's (1972) earlier notation. Here, the dependent variable, say dental contact, is predicted by a set of dummy variables representing the age, period, and cohort effects. Expressed in mathematical notation in Equation 1.3, this approach takes the following form:

$$Y = k + \sum_{i=1}^{I-1} a_i A_i + \sum_{j=1}^{J-1} p_j P_j + \sum_{k=1}^{K-1} c_k C_k + e \qquad (1.3)$$

where Y is dental contact, k is the intercept, A is the set of dummy variables representing the age categories and the a_i are their regression coefficients, P is the set of dummy variables representing the different periods and the p_j are their regression coefficients, C is the set of dummy variables representing the various birth cohorts and the c_k are their regression coefficients, and e is the error or disturbance term.

Notice that this approach begins by omitting one dummy variable from each of the age, period, and cohort parent terms. As indicated earlier, however, Equation 1.3 remains underidentified (because of the identity problem inherent in Equation 1.1) and thus cannot be

estimated. It is at this point that Mason et al. (1973) introduce the
first of two statistical restrictions involved in their accounting formula. One additional (i.e., a fourth) dummy variable, must also be
omitted. Equation 1.4 presents an example of such a restriction in
which the additional dummy variable is omitted from the set of
variables representing the age categories:

$$Y = k + \sum_{i=1}^{I-2} a_i A_i + \sum_{j=1}^{J-1} p_j P_j + \sum_{k=1}^{K-1} c_k C_k + e \quad (1.4)$$

Here, it is assumed that two of the age categories will have equivalent
behavior (i.e., that no difference will exist between them, all other
things being equal). The second statistical restriction that must be
made for Equation 1.4 to work is that the effects of age, period, and
cohort must only be additive. That is, the effects of each must be
consistent (though not necessarily linear) throughout the range of the
other two.

If both of these statistical restrictions can be made, then the accounting framework will succeed in separating the effects of age,
period, and cohort. Unfortunately, much debate exists about whether
these restrictions are realistic, and about the problems of implementing them. On the first issue, Glenn (1976, 1977, 1989) and Palmore
(1978) have convincingly argued that many theoretical reasons exist
not to assume that age, period, and cohort always have only additive
effects. Consider, for example, the preceding discussion of the understandable interaction between age and period shown in Table 1.1. On
the second issue, Rodgers (1982a, 1982b) has demonstrated that
(a) the commission of even small errors in selecting the "right" fourth
dummy variable to be excluded can substantially alter the obtained
regression coefficients, and (b) measurement error can lead to highly
inaccurate estimates of the regression coefficients even when the
"precisely correct" fourth dummy variable is excluded.

Even if the two statistical restrictions can be reasonably and accurately made, however, the accounting framework is only a statistical
technique (see Hertzog & Schaie, 1982; Schaie & Hertzog, 1982,
1985). It can only estimate the differences between age-groups, periods, and cohorts. The accounting framework, in and of itself, cannot
explain why such differences exist. To explain what the estimated
differences mean requires a clearly formulated theoretical framework
that a priori specifies one's expectations for the data. Thus, despite
the considerable attention given to cohort analytic methods during
the past two decades, much remains to be done.

Indeed, after reviewing all of the statistical methods (including the accounting framework) that have been developed for the purpose of separating age, period, and cohort effects, Kupper, Janis, Karmous, & Greenberg (1985) are less than sanguine about the utility of such techniques. They (1985) conclude that:

> . . . the statistical analysis of APC data is plagued by many unresolved issues and potential sources of error. . . . Given these . . . it is our position that such regression methods cannot be said to provide important interpretational advantages over traditional graphical [or standard cohort table] approaches. (pp.-826–827)

Thus, it is advisable that any cohort analysis begin with the visual inspection of standard cohort tables (or graphs), and proceed to more sophisticated statistical techniques like the accounting framework only after any patterns revealed from the simpler methods have been clearly appreciated.

OVERVIEW OF WHAT IS TO COME

The remainder of this book is divided into five chapters. Each serves a specific and important purpose in the presentation of the study. Although they are sequenced to build one upon another, they are sufficiently independent to facilitate the reader who desires to proceed directly to any chapter of particular interest. Nonetheless, it would likely be beneficial to read Chapter 3 before taking up the results of any of the regression-based cohort analyses.

Chapter 2 provides an overview of what we do and do not know about the elderly's use of health services. It contains two major sections. The first is an epidemiological assessment that focuses on the heterogeneity that exists. The second is a discussion of the methodological issues involved in studying health and the use of health services.

The design, methods, and data used in the study are the subject of Chapter 3. It begins with the presentation, elaboration, and justification of the eight-cohort-by-four-survey design. This is followed by a detailed overview of the behavioral model and the regression-based cohort analytic techniques. Chapter 3 concludes with a description of the HISs, and of the operationalization of the independent and dependent variables.

Chapter 4 contains the results of applying the traditional cohort analysis techniques to all of the measures of health and health behavior. This includes the analysis of health status, and the measures of informal and formal use of health services. Chapter 5 presents results of the regression-based cohort analyses. This includes the analysis of health status, and the measures of formal and informal use of health services. Finally, chapter 6 presents the conclusions that can be drawn from both the traditional and regression-based cohort analyses, as well as the implications that they have for public policy concerning the health and health care of elderly Americans.

REFERENCES

Achenbaum, A. (1985). Societal views of the aged. In R. Binstock & E. Shanas (Eds.), *Handbook of aging and the social sciences* (2nd ed.) (pp. 129–148). New York: Van Nostrand Reinhold.

Aday, L. A., Fleming, G. V., & Andersen, R. M. (1984). *Access to medical care in the U.S.: Who has it, who doesn't?* Chicago: Pluribus Press.

Anderson, O. W. (1985). *Health services in the United Sates: A growth enterprise since 1875.* Ann Arbor: Health Administration Press.

Baltes, P. B. (1968). Longitudinal and cross-sectional sequences in the study of age and generation effects. *Human Development, 11,* 145–171.

Banting, D. W. (1984). Dental caries in the elderly. *Gerodontology, 3,* 55–67.

Beck, J. (1984). The epidemiology of dental diseases in the elderly. *Gerodontology, 3,* 5–15.

Binstock, R. H. (1985). The oldest-old: A fresh perspective or compassionate ageism revisited. *Milbank Memorial Fund Quarterly, 63,* 420–451.

Binstock, R. H., & Kahana, J. (1988). An essay on—*Setting limits: Medical goals in an aging society. The Gerontologist, 28,* 424–426.

Birren, J. B., & Cunningham, W. (1985). Research on the psychology of aging: Principles, concepts, and theory. In J. Birren & K. W. Schaie (Eds.), *Handbook of the psychology of aging* (2nd ed.) (pp. 3–34). New York: Van Nostrand Reinhold.

Birren, J., & Renner, V. J. (1977). Research on the psychology of aging. In J. Birren & K. W. Schaie (Eds.), *Handbook of psychology of aging* (pp. 3–38). New York: Van Nostrand Reinhold.

Botwinick, J. (1977). *Aging and behavior.* New York: Springer Publishing Co.

Brody, E. M. (1985). Parent care as normative family stress. *The Gerontologist, 25,* 19–29.

Butler, R. N. (1975). *Why survive: Being old in America.* New York: Harper & Row.

Callahan, D. (1987). *Setting limits: Medical goals in an aging society.* New York: Simon & Schuster.

Cape, R. D., Coe, R. M., & Rossman, I. (Eds.). (1983). *Fundamentals of geriatric medicine.* New York: Raven Press.

Cohn, R. (1972). Mathematical Note. In M. Riley, M. Johnson, & A. Foner, (Eds.), *Aging and Society: Volume Three: A Sociology of Age Stratification* (pp. 85–88). New York: Russell Sage Foundation.

Comfort, A. (1956). *The biology of senescence.* London: Routledge, Kegan, & Paul.

Conrad, D. A. (1982). Dental care demand: Age specific estimates for the 65 years and older population. *Health Care Financing Review, 4,* 47–56.

Cornoni-Huntley, J. C., Ostfeld, A. M., Taylor, J. A., & Wallace, R. B. (1986). *Establishment of populations for epidemiologic study of the elderly: Study design and methodology* (DHHS Publication No. 87-1234). Washington, DC: Government Printing Office.

Cowdry, E. V. (1942). *Problems in ageing*. Baltimore: Williams & Wilkins.

Dement, W., Richardson, G., Prinz, P. Carskadon, M., Kripke, D., Czeisler, C. (1985). Changes of sleep and wakefulness with age. In C. Finch & E. Schneider (Eds.), *Handbook of the biology of aging* (2nd ed.) (pp. 692-720). New York: Van Nostrand Reinhold.

Department of Health and Human Services. (1982). *Third report to the president and the Congress on the status of health professions personnel in the United States* (DHHS Publication No. 82-2). Washington, DC: Government Printing Office.

Elder, G. H. (1974). *Children of the great depression*. Chicago: University of Chicago Press.

Elder, G. H. (1975). Age differentiation and the life course. *Annual Review of Sociology, 1,* 165-190.

Elder, G. H., & Liker, J. K. (1982). Hard times in women's lives: Historical influences across 40 years. *American Journal of Sociology, 88,* 241-269.

Estes, C. (1988, August). *Biomedicalization of aging: Dilemmas and dangers*. Paper presented to the annual meeting of the American Sociological Association, Atlanta, GA.

Evashwick, C. J., Conrad, D. A., & Lee, F. (1982). Factors related to utilization of dental services by the elderly. *American Journal of Public Health, 72,* 1129-1135.

Fetter, R. B., Shin, Y., Freeman, J. L., Averill, R. F., & Thompson, J. D. (1980). Case mix definition by diagnosis-related groups. *Medical Care, 18*(Suppl. 2), 1-53.

Fienberg, S. E., & Mason, W. M. (1978). Identification and estimation of age-period-cohort models in the analysis of discrete archival data. *Sociological Methodology, 1980,* 1-67.

Finch, C. E., & Schneider, E. L. (Eds.). (1985). *Handbook of the biology of aging* (2nd ed.). New York: Van Nostrand Reinhold.

Fischer, D. (1977). *Growing old in America* (rev. ed.). New York: Oxford University Press.

Glenn, N. D. (1976). Cohort analysts' futile quest: Statistical attempts to separate age, period, and cohort effects. *American Sociological Review, 41,* 900-904.

Glenn, N. D. (1977). *Cohort analysis*. Beverly Hills: Sage Publications.

Glenn, N. D. (1989). A flawed approach to solving the identification problem in the estimation of mobility effect models: A comment on Brody and McRae. *Social Forces, 67,* 789-795.

Gribbin, K., Schaie, K. W., & Parham, I. A. (1980). Complexity of life style and maintenance of intellectual abilities. *Journal of Social Issues, 36,* 47-61.

Haug, M. (1981). Age and medical care utilization patterns. *Journal of Gerontology, 36,* 103-111.

Hertzog, C., & Schaie, K. W. (1982, December). *On the analysis of sequential data in life-span developmental research*. Paper presented at the annual meeting of the American Psychological Association, Washington, D.C.

Hertzog, C., Schaie, K. W., & Gribbin, K. (1978). Cardiovascular disease and changes in intellectual functioning from middle to old age. *Journal of Gerontology, 33,* 872-883.

Hogan, D. P. (1981). *Transitions and social change*. New York: Academic Press.

Kiyak, A. (1984). Age differences in oral health and beliefs. *Journal of Public Health Dentistry, 42,* 404–412.

Kiyak, A. (1987). An explanatory model of older persons' use of dental services: Implications for health policy. *Medical Care, 25,* 936–951.

Knoke, D., & Hout, M. (1976). Social and demographic factors in American political party affiliations, 1952–72. *American Sociological Review, 39,* 700–713.

Kupper, L. W., Janis, J. M., Karmous, A., & Greenberg, B. G. (1985). Statistical Age-Period-Cohort Analysis: A Review and Critique. *Journal of Chronic Disease 38,* 811–830.

Labouvie-Vief, G. (1985). Intelligence and cognition. In J. Birren & W. Schaie (Eds.), *Handbook of the psychology of aging* (2nd ed.) (pp. 500–530). New York: Van Nostrand Reinhold.

Lewis-Beck, M. (1980). *Applied regression analysis.* Beverly Hills: Sage Publications.

Linton, R. (1936). *Study of man.* New York: Appleton-Century.

Lyman, K. (1988, August). *Bringing the social back in: A critique of the medicalization of dementia.* Paper presented at the annual meeting of the American Sociological Association, Atlanta, GA.

McRae, J. A., & Brody, C. J. (1989). Reply to Glenn. *Social Forces, 67,* 796–798.

Maddox, G. L. (1979). Sociology of later life. *Annual Review of Sociology, 5,* 113–135.

Maddox, G. L., & Campbell, R. T. (1985). Scope, concepts, and methods in the study of aging. In R. H. Binstock & E. Shanas (Eds.), *Handbook of aging and the social sciences* (2nd ed.) (pp. 3–34). New York: Van Nostrand Reinhold.

Mason, W. H., & Fienberg, S. E. (Eds.). (1984). *Cohort analysis in social research: Beyond the identification problem.* New York: Springer-Verlag.

Mason, K. O., Mason, W. M., Winsborough, H. H., & Poole, W. K. (1973). Some methodological issues in cohort analysis of archival data. *American Sociological Review, 38,* 242–258.

Mason, K. O., Mason, W. M., Winsborough, H. H., & Poole, W. K. (1976). Reply to Glenn. *American Sociological Review, 41,* 904–905.

McKinlay, J. M. (1985, September). *Health care utilization by the elderly: Special considerations, methodological developments, and theoretical issues.* Paper presented at invitational workshop on Aging and Formal Health Care. Jointly sponsored by the National Institute on Aging and the National Center for Health Services Research, Bethesda, MD.

Mechanic, D. (1988). Illness behavior and medical care use by the elderly. In M. Ory & K. Bond (Eds.), *Aging and the use of formal care* (pp. 244–255). New York: Tavistock Publications.

Mossey, J. M., Havens, B., & Wolinsky, F. D. (1988). The consistency of formal health care utilization. In M. Ory & K. Bond (Eds.), *Aging and the use of formal care* (pp. 81–98). New York: Tavistock Publications.

Mossey, J. M., & Shapiro, E. (1985). Physician use by the elderly over an eight-year period. *American Journal of Public Health, 75,* 1333–1334.

Palmore, E. (1978). When can age, period, and cohort be separated? *Social Forces, 57,* 285–295.

Parsons, T. (1951). *The social system.* New York: Free Press.

Polissar, L., & Diehr, P. K. (1982). Regression analysis in health services research: The use of dummy variables. *Medical Care, 20,* 959–974.

Pomper, F. (1976). *The voter's choice.* New York: Dodd, Mead.

Riley, M. W. (1972). The succession of cohorts. In M. Riley, M. Johnson, &

A. Foner (Eds.), *Aging and society: A sociology of age stratification* (Vol. 3) (pp. 515–582). New York: Russell Sage.

Riley, M. W. (1973). Aging and cohort succession: Interpretations and misinterpretations. *Public Opinion Quarterly, 37,* 35–49.

Riley, M. W. (1976). Age strata in social systems. In R. Binstock & E. Shanas (Eds.), *Handbook of aging and the social sciences* (pp. 189–217). New York: Van Nostrand Reinhold.

Riley, M. W. (1981). Health behavior of older people: Toward a new paradigm. In D. Parron, F. Solomon, & J. Rodin (Eds.), *Health, behavior, and aging* (pp. 25–39). Washington, DC: National Academy Press.

Riley, M. W. (1985). Age strata in social systems. In R. Binstock & E. Shanas (Eds.), *Handbook of aging and the social sciences* (2nd ed.) (pp. 369–411). New York: Van Nostrand Reinhold.

Riley, M. W. (1987). On the significance of age in sociology. *American Sociological Review, 52,* 1–14.

Riley, M. W., Foner, A., Moore, M. E., Hess, B. B., & Roth, B. K. (1968). *Aging and society: An inventory of research findings* (Vol. 1). New York: Russell Sage.

Riley, M. W., Foner, A., & Waring, J. (1988). Sociology of age. In N. J. Smelser (Ed.), *Handbook of sociology* (pp. 243–290). Newbury Park, CA: Sage Publications.

Riley, M. W., Johnson, M., & Foner, A. (Eds.). (1972). *Aging and society: A sociology of age stratification* (Vol. 3). New York: Russell Sage.

Rodgers, W. L. (1982a). Estimable functions of age, period, and cohort effects. *American Sociological Review, 47,* 774–787.

Rodgers, W. L. (1982b). Reply to Mason, Smith, and Fienberg. *American Sociological Review, 47,* 793–796.

Rosenwaike, I. (1985). A demographic portrait of the oldest old. *Milbank Memorial Fund Quarterly, 63,* 187–205.

Rosow, I. (1985). Status and role change through the life cycle. In R. Binstock & E. Shanas (Eds.), *Handbook of aging and the social sciences* (2nd ed.) (pp. 62–93). New York: Van Nostrand Reinhold.

Ryder, N. B. (1965). The cohort as a concept in the study of social change. *American Sociological Review, 30,* 843–861.

Schaie, K. W. (1965). A general model for the study of developmental problems. *Psychological Bulletin, 64,* 92–107.

Schaie, K. W. (1981). Psychological changes from midlife to old age: Implications for the maintenance of mental health. *American Journal of Orthopsychiatry, 51,* 199–218.

Schaie, K. W. (1984). Midlife influences upon intellectual functioning in old age. *International Journal of Behavioral Development, 7,* 463–478.

Schaie, K. W., & Hertzog, C. (1983). Fourteen-year cohort-sequential studies of adult intelligence. *Developmental Psychology, 19,* 531–543.

Schaie, K. W., & Hertzog, C. (1985). Measurement in the psychology of adulthood and aging. In J. Birren & W. Schaie (Eds.), *Handbook of the psychology of aging* (2nd ed.) (pp. 61–94). New York: Van Nostrand Reinhold.

Schaie, K. W., & Hertzog, C. (1986). Toward a comprehensive model of adult intellectual development: Contributions of the Seattle Longitudinal Study. *Advances in Human Intelligence, 3,* 79–118.

Schaie, K. W., Labouvie, G., & Buech, B. U. (1973). Generational and cohort-specific differences in adult cognitive functioning: A fourteen-year study of independent samples. *Developmental Psychology*, *9*, 151–156.

Smith, H. L., Mason, W. M., & Fienberg, S. E. (1982). More chimeras of the age-period-cohort accounting framework: Comments on Rodgers. *American Sociological Review*, *47*, 787–793.

Torrens, P. R. (1984). Historical evolution and overview of health services in the United States. In S. Williams & P. Torrens (Eds.), *Introduction to health services* (2nd ed.) (pp. 1–25). New York: John Wiley & Sons.

Torrey, B. B. (1985). Sharing increasing costs on declining income: The visible dilemma of the invisible aged. *Milbank Memorial Fund Quarterly*, *63*, 377–394.

Van Gennep, A. (1908). *Rites of passage*. Chicago: University of Chicago Press.

Wan, T. T. H. (1988). Antecedents of health services utilization in the older population. In M. Ory & K. Bond (Eds.), *Aging and the use of formal care* (pp. 52–78). New York: Tavistock Publications.

White, T. N. (1961). *The making of the president, 1960*. New York: Simon & Schuster.

Wolinsky, F. D. (1988). *The sociology of health: Principles, practitioners, and issues* (2nd ed.). Belmont: Wadsworth Publishing.

Wolinsky, F. D., & Arnold, C. L. (1989). A birth cohort analysis of dental contact among elderly Americans. *American Journal of Public Health*, *79*, 47–51.

Wolinsky, F. D., Arnold, C. L., & Nallapati, I. V. (1988). Explaining the declining rate of physician utilization among the oldest-old. *Medical Care*, *26*, 544–553.

Wolinsky, F. D., & Coe, R. M. (1984). Physician and hospital utilization among noninstitutionalized elderly adults: An analysis of the health interview survey. *Journal of Gerontology*, *39*, 334–341.

Wolinsky, F. D., Coe, R. M., Miller, D. K., Prendergast, J. M., Creel, M. J., & Chavez, M. N. (1983). Health services utilization among the noninstitutionalized elderly. *Journal of Health and Social Behavior*, *24*, 325–337.

Wolinsky, F. D., Mosely, R. R., & Coe, R. M. (1986). A cohort analysis of the use of health services by elderly Americans. *Journal of Health and Social Behavior*, *27*, 209–219.

Chapter 2

What We Do
and Do Not Know

It is often said, by both the public and policy makers, that older Americans are in poorer health and use more health services than their younger counterparts. When speaking in terms of statistical averages, this is quite correct (Department of Health and Human Services, 1988). The repetitive presentation (since the 1960s) of such statistical evidence, like per capita health care expenses, as well as the selective use of vignettes describing sick and needy individuals, has led to the development of a class-based conception of the elderly (Binstock, 1985). This conception asserts that great homogeneity exists in the elderly's health and health behavior (Neugarten, 1974). That, however, is simply not the case (Wolinsky & Arnold, 1988).

Indeed, for more than a decade gerontologists interested in health and health behavior have called for the recognition of the heterogeneity that exists in these areas (e.g., Bloom & Soper, 1980; Butler, 1975; Evashwick, Rowe, Diehr, & Branch, 1984; Haug, 1981; Kovar, 1977, 1986; Shanas & Maddox, 1985; Soldo & Manton, 1985; Wan & Arling, 1983; Wolinsky & Coe, 1984). A thoughtful examination of the most recent federal government publication on the subject supports their call (Havlik et al., 1987). It is the purpose of this chapter, then, to provide the reader with an overview of what we do and do not know about the elderly's health and health behavior. In so doing, special emphasis will be placed on the heterogeneity issue.

To accomplish these tasks the present chapter is divided into two major sections. The first provides an epidemiological overview of the elderly's health and their use of health services. It begins with a discussion of the latent assumption of homogeneity in the literature, including as illustrative examples the use of limited age, living arrangement, and ethnicity categorizations. Then, the trend toward the heterogeneity perspective is reviewed including such matters as differentiating heavy from moderate from low users of services, and examining the consistency of their patterns of use over time. The first section concludes by presenting evidence of the differential health and use of health services across various age and ethnic groups taken from a pooled analysis of the HISs.

The second section of the chapter focuses on methodological issues in studying health and use of health services. It begins with a focus on measurement issues, including the differences in meaning and interpretation between objective versus subjective measures of health status, and between contact, volume, episode, and recency measures of the use of health services. Modeling issues are considered next including the differences between categorical versus metric analyses, limited versus saturated models, and the functional forms of various predictive equation systems. To illustrate the importance of these issues for public policy recommendations, this section concludes with a multivariate analysis of health and health behavior, using the data taken from the pooled HISs once again.

THE EPIDEMIOLOGY OF DIFFERENTIAL HEALTH AND USE OF HEALTH SERVICES

In beginning her landmark paper, which was directed toward a public health and not a gerontological audience, Kovar (1977) eloquently addressed the homogeneity assumption head-on:

> It would be a mistake to think of the elderly as a homogeneous population. As a group, they are more likely than younger persons to suffer from multiple, chronic, often permanent conditions that may be disabling, but the majority are living active lives—many of them in their own households. The range in health status is just as great in this age group as in any other, even though the proportion of persons who have health problems increases with age and a minor

health problem that might be quickly alleviated at younger ages tends to linger. Aging is a process that continues over the entire lifespan at differing rates among different persons. The rate of aging varies among populations and among individuals in the same population. It varies even within an individual because different body systems do not age at the same rate. (p. 9)

Kovar's observations underscore the paradox in which gerontologists studying the health and illness behavior of the elderly have for so long themselves been ageist, albeit unintentionally so, toward their subjects. If Binstock (1985) is correct, the increasing focus on the oldest-old (i.e., those 85 years of age and older) that has been stimulated in part by the National Institute on Aging (via major, special funding programs [see Suzman & Riley, 1985; Suzman & Willis, 1988]) may actually intensify the problem. Binstock fears that the data now coming to light on the oldest-old will result in new stereotypes that serve only to generate and reinforce anxieties about age-group conflicts over the allocation of health services. As two notable examples, consider the increasing popularity of the phrase "intergenerational equity" in discussions about the economic implications of the rising dependency ratio, and the growing ethical debate on what society "ought" to be expected to do for the very old (Callahan, 1987).

Age Homogeneity Assumption

How did this problem get its start? It probably began with the enactment of the enabling legislation for Social Security, which somewhat arbitrarily established a chronological age marker for eligibility. Ever since, largely because of the power of inertia, a tendency has existed to characterize the elderly as that apparently homogeneous group of persons aged 65 years or more. This makes one wonder how different gerontology and geriatrics would be had that enabling legislation specified an age percentile marker for eligibility. In 1930 age 65 marked the 95th percentile in the age distribution. By 1986, however, the chronological age that marked the 95th percentile had risen to age 75.

From the health and health behavior perspective, the homogeneity assumption appears to have been somewhat tacitly accepted in much of the literature before the early 1970s. By then the changing demographic dynamics had resulted in an increasing number of persons older than age 65 who were healthy, active, and clearly not wards of the state. This, of course, diminished the analytic utility of the term "elderly." Rather than accept outright the heterogeneity of the elderly population, gerontologists embraced Neugarten's (1974) suggestion that a new distinction be made between the young-old and the old-old, in which the latter embodied the traditional characterizations of the "elderly."

Unfortunately, too many gerontologists failed to grasp Neugarten's main point, and simply began to compare and contrast the two age groups (see Snider, 1980). That is, they merely cut the deck of elderly individuals into two piles. The reasons lie in the immaturity of the field, its descriptive rather than analytic orientation, and convenience. In any event, the result has been only a subtle shift in the adherence to the homogeneity assumption from studying the health and illness behavior of the elderly to comparing and contrasting it between the young-old and the old-old, and, now, to comparing and contrasting it between the young-old, the old-old, and the oldest-old.

Even when other factors have been introduced to account for the within-groups variance in health and health behavior, the focus (despite the claims of Shanas and Maddox [1985] to the contrary) has been more on recutting the deck along another dimension (as in a limited, contingency table approach), rather than on recognizing the underlying heterogeneity of individuals. For example, consider the manner in which living arrangements and ethnicity have been introduced. Regarding the former, it has generally been assumed that elderly individuals who live alone are more likely to view themselves to be in poorer health and to use more health services than their counterparts who live with others. Various reasons are given, all of which relate to the broad theme of social supports including its emotional, instrumental, and affirmational dimensions (see Antonucci, 1985; Krause, 1988). A growing body of evidence exists that not only substantiates these claims but also views the effects of widowhood to be spurious to those of living arrangements (see Homan, Haddock, Winner, Coe, & Wolinsky, 1986; Cafferata, 1987).

Where, however, has the introduction of living arrangements into the study of health and health behavior led us? Unfortunately, it has only introduced another dichotomous factor (living alone vs. with others) with which to cut the deck. It has not focused attention on the more important conceptual issue, which involves the dynamics of change in the convoy of social support over the life course (Antonucci & Akiyama, 1987; Kahn, 1979; Kahn & Antonucci, 1980), and their effects on health and health behavior. Indeed, all of these studies make the simplifying assumption that current living arrangements are both stable, and are the cause (rather than the effect) of social support levels and their sequelae. The end result is that the spirit (if not the letter) of the homogeneity assumption remains fundamentally intact.

The introduction of ethnicity to the study of health and health behavior has also been a relatively recent phenomenon, despite long-standing evidence in the social sciences of its critical importance (Jackson, 1967). Indeed, Jackson (1985) has been reluctant to review comprehensively the ethnogerontological literature because of its "largely descriptive and inconclusive nature" (p. 264). The typical treatment of ethnicity initially involved a focus on white subjects, avoiding the issue altogether by excluding nonwhites from the analysis. This approach explicitly assumed whites to be culturally homogeneous and implicitly assumed nonwhites to be different yet homogeneous as well.

During the late 1960s to early 1970s the exclusion of nonwhite subjects from the study of health and the use of health services was recognized by gerontologists as too limiting, and a new approach emerged. This awareness of the unsatisfactory exclusion of nonwhites resulted in the reliance on an equally unsatisfactory racially based dichotomization, with whites compared and contrasted with blacks, and nonwhite-nonblack individuals excluded from the analysis (see Jackson [1985] for a detailed review). By the late 1970s the increasing interest in the Hispanic subpopulation resulted in the expansion of the racially based dichotomy into a racially based trichotomy: whites, blacks, and Hispanics. Unfortunately, the implicit assumption of homogeneity within each of the three groups continued, despite substantial evidence for the existence of cultural heterogeneity (especially within the Hispanic group [cf., Anderson, Lewis, Giachello, Aday, & Chiu, 1981]). Indeed, even Jackson (1985) ultimately falls into the Hispanic homogeneity trap, assuming the cultural diversity within this group to be relatively unimportant.

Most recently several investigators have made pleas to disaggregate the Hispanic category, at least into its own tripartite division of Puerto Rican Americans, Cuban Americans, and Mexican Americans (Schur, Bernstein, & Berk, 1987; Travino & Moss, 1984; Report of the Secretary's Task Force on Black and Minority Health, 1985). These authors argue that more (albeit unidentified) cultural heterogeneity than homogeneity exists among Hispanics, and that this in turn results in different patterns of health and use of health services. The evidence for the differential health behavior that they present is rather convincing. For example, Travino and Moss (1984) have shown that the annual rate of physician use ranges from a low of 6.6 among Puerto Rican elderly, to a high of 10.8 among Cuban elderly. Schur et al. (1987) have shown that among those with a usual source of care, 83.2% of Cubans receive their care in a doctor's office compared with 48.9% of Puerto Ricans.

Despite the advances that this disaggregation of the Hispanic group provides for our understanding of the health and health behavior of the elderly, it really only serves to cut the deck into a few more piles. That is, it does not further our understanding of ethnically related cultural differences. Rather, it merely subdivides what was once considered to be one homogeneous Hispanic subpopulation into three different but presumably internally homogeneous subpopulations. It is important to note that this is done not on the basis of theory but on the convenience of national origin in the data. It is the heterogeneity within each of these Hispanic subpopulations that needs to be explained, perhaps by the introduction of measures of ethnic identification or self-conception (see Saenz & Aquirre, 1988).

These three illustrations (i.e., limited age, living arrangements, and ethnicity characterizations) make the point. Research that takes heterogeneity explicitly into account has come about only in the past two decades. Moreover, despite growing evidence and logic to the contrary, the latent homogeneity assumption has not yet been cast off effectively. Rather, what has emerged is somewhat analogous to a "risk factor mentality" in which limited categorical factors (also including sex, education, and economic status [Federal Council on Aging, 1981]) are introduced in an epidemiological fashion in the hope of identifying a few subpopulations, each of which is relatively homogeneous in its health and health behavior. In so doing, the spirit (if not the letter) of the latent homogeneity assumption lives on.

Emergence of a Different Perspective

Perhaps among the clearer and more recent challenges to the homogeneity assumption are the growing reliance on multivariate analytic techniques, and the application to the elderly of conceptual and empirical models developed for the nonelderly. The former more explicitly recognizes the heterogeneity of health and health behavior within the elderly population, and the latter sets that heterogeneity among the elderly on a par with the heterogeneity traditionally found among the nonelderly population. The results reported in the literature have demonstrated the utility of these approaches (Branch et al., 1981; Coulton & Frost, 1982; Evashwick et al., 1984; Eve, 1982,

1984; Eve & Friedsam, 1980; Haug, 1981; Russell, 1981; Stoller, 1982; Wan & Arling, 1983; Wan & Odell, 1981; Wolinsky & Coe, 1984; Wolinsky et al., 1983).

Indeed, these studies find that although health status is the most important determinant of health services use, most of the variation remains unexplained. This is consistent with the findings from comparable studies of the nonelderly population, underscoring the fact that the health and health behavior of the elderly is not more homogeneous than that of the young. To the contrary, the fact that these models explain a little less of the variation in the use of health services by the elderly, as contrasted to the nonelderly, suggests that more (not less) heterogeneity exists among older Americans.

Perhaps the most important aspect of these challenges, however, are their emphases on the conceptual and statistical elaboration of relationships. This denotes a different perspective directed more toward the explanation of the health and health behavior of elderly *individuals*, rather than on the characterization of various *subpopulations*. The importance of this new perspective can not be emphasized enough. As the number of factors included in these models increases, it becomes clear that the individual is *the* critical ingredient in the analysis. Indeed, the growing number of factors underscores the importance of individual differentiation. Although one can (erroneously) assume that certain social groups are homogeneous in some aspect of their behavior, that same assumption cannot be made for individuals.

Unfortunately, the differentiation issue is not as straightforward as it may seem. Limits exist on how far one can go in the pursuit of modeling heterogeneity. Technically, constraints are imposed by the available degrees of freedom. These technical limitations, however, are easily enough overcome by the reliance on large-scale surveys. It is the conceptual constraints that are actually the most limiting. The purpose of statistical analysis, after all, is to reveal and summarize shared patterns of behavior in the data. Therefore, it is impossible to avoid some amount of aggregation (and typing) if we are to reveal and summarize those shared patterns of behavior. Ultimately, then, one is left with optimizing the trade-off between statistical aggregation and individual assessment. It should be clear from the preceding discussion that, to date, research on the aged's health and use of health services has erred on the side of aggregation.

Two more focused issues concerning the health and health behavior of the elderly have surfaced during the 1980s that have also explicitly confronted the homogeneity assumption, albeit in a different way. These issues involve the recognition that a continuum exists of the amount of health services used by elderly individuals that ranges from heavy to moderate to low, and the examination of the consistency of the use patterns of elderly individuals over time. Work on the former is important for two reasons. One is that standard predictive models of the use of health services have been shown to fare more poorly when heavy users (defined as those above the 95th percentile in the distribution) are included in the analysis without adjustment, as opposed to when their use levels are artificially constrained to be more moderate (i.e., truncated at the 95th percentile; see Wolinsky & Coe, 1984). This suggests that both the reasons for and their priority of importance in determining the use of health services differ between heavy and nonheavy users. Those differences have salient implications for the study of health and health behavior including the possibility that (a) all use of health services by heavy users is fundamentally nondiscretionary (i.e., disease, physician, or delivery system generated, and appropriately so), and therefore (b) health education and cost-containment efforts directed at both heavy users and their providers is not likely to be successful.

The other reason why the identification of heavy users is important focuses on disconfirming the homogeneity assumption among the elderly by establishing that the basis for heavy users' homogeneity is not age. In a remarkable examination of the 1980 National Medical Care Utilization and Expenditure Survey, Berki et al. (1986) classified separately high, low, and moderate users of hospital, physician, and prescription drug services. Berki et al. (1986) found that:

> Both univariate and multivariable analyses [of all ages combined] show that the most important distinguishing characteristics of high users of any of the three medical services are poor health status, severe functional limitations, and the presence of multiple medical conditions—most importantly cancer, cardiac disorders, musculo-skeletal diseases, respiratory diseases, and injuries and poisonings. Almost all high-volume users of every service category (88 percent for hospital days, 89 percent for ambulatory visits, and 94 percent for prescribed medications) had at least three different diagnostic conditions reported during the year. (p. 1)

Thus, it is not the elderly per se who are high users of health services, but those with multiple and severe health problems (see also Kovar, 1986).

Berki et al. (1986) also demonstrated what a remarkably small segment of the noninstitutionalized population belongs to the high-users classification, and how much health care costs for this group.

High users of hospital care represent 1.7% of the population but account for 54.4% of those requiring hospital stays; high users of ambulatory services represent 4.5% of the population but account for 32.3% of all those making ambulatory visits; and high users of prescription drugs represent 5.9% of the population but account for 32.9% of all those acquiring prescriptions. At the other end of the extreme, for example, low users of health services represent 17% of the population but account for only 3.3% of all those making ambulatory visits.

Clearly, then, heavy users represent the greatest drain on the health care delivery system. Besides being severely ill, however, who are these heavy users? More often than not, they are people in the process of dying. Indeed, Lubitz and Prihoda (1983) have shown that a large proportion of Medicare expenditures occur during the recipient's last year of life. As a result, the heavy-user issue was initially viewed as an aging problem because it emerged from analyses of Medicare expenditure data, and the elderly have higher mortality rates. Recently, however, Roos, Montgomery, and Roos (1987) have taken the issue a step further by using data from the Manitoba Longitudinal Study of Aging to disentangle the effects of aging from those of dying. They (Roos et al., 1987) conclude that:

> In Manitoba as in the United States, hospital utilization markedly increases in a short period before death, dying has a greater impact on utilization than age per se, and small numbers of individuals consume a disproportionate amount of care. Also . . . very elderly decedents spend somewhat fewer days in [the] hospital and make fewer physician visits than those dying at younger ages. . . . [Thus] the time between onset of illness and death may be shorter for older decedents. (p. 253)

Moreover, Roos et al. (1987) found a substantial number of individuals in all age-groups, including the elderly, whose deaths did not result in significant health care expenditures. Therefore, the homogeneity assumption fails to apply even to the special case of the dying elderly (see also Kovar, 1986).

The intriguing combination of high health care costs and marked heterogeneity in use patterns among the elderly has focused interest on a related issue. Over time, do consistently high or low users of health services exist, and, if so, how might they be characterized? Because this question can only be addressed by using data from large-scale, longitudinal surveys, no definitive answers are presently available (Mossey, Havens, & Wolinsky, 1988). Nonetheless, preliminary reports from the Manitoba study (Mossey & Shapiro, 1985) indicate that about 60% of the noninstitutionalized elderly, including both those who were alive at the end of the study and those who died during it, were rather consistent (i.e., within four visits, annually) in their use of physician services for 6 or more of the 8 years of data collection. Moreover, even though more of the decedents had consistently high rates of physician use (seven or more visits annually) as compared to the survivors (21.5% vs. 14.2%), an equivalent proportion of them (about 20%) were consistently very low users (zero to two visits) even during their last year of life. Thus, these data suggest that a relatively small proportion of the elderly are consistently heavy users of heath services.

Who, however, are these consistent users? Using multivariate logistic regression analyses and standard indicators taken from the behavioral model of the use of health services (Andersen, 1968), Mossey et al. (1988) were unable to differentiate consistent from inconsistent users. They were, however, able to discriminate between levels of use among the consistent users. The need for health care (measured by the illness scale [see Mossey & Roos, 1987]) accounted for 54% of the variance among the survivors and 63% of the variance among the decedents. All of the other factors combined added less than 4% to the explained variance. Indeed, the effect of age was not statistically significant among the survivors, and it had only a marginal (and negative) effect among the decedents. As a result, Mossey et al. (1988) conclude that consistently high use reflects ill health, and consistently low use reflects good health, period.

When taken together, these studies of heavy versus nonheavy and consistent versus inconsistent users of health services make a most important point. Sufficiently compelling evidence exists to drive gerontologists away from their traditional reliance on chronological age as an important, if not the most important, factor in their research. As a variable, age simply has limited predictive utility for the analysis of data on health and the use of health services. Failure to recognize and comprehend the implications of this limited explanatory power only serves to maintain the latent homogeneity assumption artificially.

Evidence of Heterogeneity of Health and Use of Health Services

This section concludes with a review of the empirical evidence demonstrating the differential health and use of health services among the elderly. Because of the increasing availability of comprehensive data on the elderly in general (see Havlik et al., 1987), and on the oldest-old in particular (see Cornoni-Huntley, et al. 1985), only a brief overview of the health and health behavior data available from pooling individuals aged 45 years or older from the 1976 to 1985 HISs is presented. The HISs were pooled to provide a sufficient number of cases for stable parameter estimates within various subpopulations.

Table 2.1 contains, by various age-groups (for comparative purposes), the percentage reporting their health to be excellent or good, the percentage with chronic conditions causing limitations in everyday activities, the percentage with 1 or more days of restricted activity because of health reasons during the preceding 2 weeks, the percentage with 1 or more days of bed disability owing to health reasons during the preceding 2 weeks, the percentage having one or more physician visits during the preceding year the number of physician visits during the preceding year, (among those with doctor visits), the percentage having one or more hospital episodes during the preceding year, the number of nights spent in the hospital during the preceding year (among those with hospital episodes), and the percentage having one or more visits to a dentist during the preceding year.

As expected, a perfectly consistent, monotonic pattern exists when age (columnar) comparisons are made for all four health-status measures. The older the age-group, the poorer the average health status. Similarly as expected, a generally consistent pattern exists when age comparisons are made for the five measures of health services use. The older the age-group, the higher the average use of health services. The two exceptions involve physician and dental contact. For the former, only the oldest-old break the pattern, with their physician contact rates dropping off by about 2%. This is consistent with previous reports (see Soldo & Manton, 1985; Wolinsky, Arnold, & Nallapati, 1988; Wolinsky, Mosely, & Coe, 1986), suggesting the possibility of the onset of a significant alteration of health behavior among octogenarians and nonagenarians. The dental contact rates monotonically decline across age groups. This, too, is consistent with previous reports. It has, however, recently been shown to be the result of cohort succession rather than an effect of the aging process (see Wolinsky & Arnold, 1989).

Because of the large number of cases, all of the differences shown in Table 2.1 are statistically significant well beyond conventional probability levels. This should not, however, be taken as support for an age-graded homogeneity assumption. To underscore that fact, Table 2.2 shows comparable data broken down further by sex and ethnicity. As

Table 2.1 Health and Use of Health Services Data by Age-Group*

Age group	% in excellent or good health	% limited activity days	% restricted activity days	% bed disability days	% physician contact	Average number of physician visits	% hospital contact	Average number of hospital nights	% with dental contact
65 & older	68.3	43.1	15.8	7.1	79.6	5.15	18.6	9.08	40.2
45-54	82.6	18.5	12.3	6.2	71.8	4.07	10.8	7.49	64.3
55-64	74.0	29.5	14.3	6.5	74.9	4.58	12.8	8.20	57.3
65-74	69.0	39.4	15.1	6.6	78.9	5.04	16.9	8.97	44.7
75-84	67.1	46.7	16.8	7.6	81.4	5.36	21.0	9.18	34.3
85 & older	66.9	62.0	17.4	9.9	79.6	5.21	23.2	9.40	22.6

*Taken from the pooled 1972, 1973, 1976, 1977, 1980, 1981, 1984, and 1985 Health Interview Surveys.

indicated, within each age group remarkable (and statistically significant) differences exist in both health and health behavior between the sexes and across the ethnic categories. Comparable breakouts based on various other factors also yield differences, as will be reflected in the multiple regression analysis of these data that concludes the next section. Thus, no doubt can exist about the heterogeneity of the health of elderly persons and their use of health services.

METHODOLOGICAL ISSUES IN STUDYING HEALTH AND USE OF HEALTH SERVICES

Although no doubt can exist about the heterogeneity of the elderly's health and their use of health services, several methodological problems limit a complete understanding of it. In general, these problems may be grouped into two categories: measurement and modeling issues. Two or three examples will suffice to illustrate each category. This section will conclude with a multiple regression analysis of the pooled HIS data demonstrating the importance of these issues for public policy.

Measurement Issues

One of the most frequently discussed measurement issues involves the distinction between objective and subjective indicators of health status. Shanas and Maddox (1985) have succinctly identified the essence of this distinction:

> In practice, health in the aged is usually defined in one of two ways: in terms of the presence or absence of disease, or in terms of how well the older person functions or his general sense of "well being." A definition of health in terms of pathology or disease states is commonly used by health personnel, particularly physicians. . . . Such a judgment is often described as "objective." . . . An alternative way to define health among the elderly is based not on pathology or disease states, but on level of functioning. . . . Thus the things that old persons can do, or think they can do, are useful indicators of both how healthy they are and the services they will require or seek. (p. 701)

Although the two approaches are not irreconcilable, neither are they isomorphic in their implications for understanding the health of elderly persons and their use of health services.

Table 2.2 Health and Use of Health Services Data by Age, Sex, and Ethnic Group*

Age, sex and ethnic group	% excellent or good health	% limited activity days	% restricted activity days	% bed disability days	% physician contact	Average no. of physician visits	% hospital contact	Average no. of hospital nights	% dental contact
AGE 45-54									
Puerto Rican (M)	73.5	27.3	17.7	12.2	70.2	5.05	13.9	8.70	45.2
Puerto Rican (F)	56.7	30.5	26.2	17.1	76.7	6.63	13.8	8.66	56.3
Cuban (M)	86.8	10.3	7.4	3.7	61.8	3.73	5.2	8.43	55.6
Cuban (F)	84.6	13.0	8.9	7.1	74.6	4.06	8.9	6.87	66.1
Mexican American (M)	77.5	14.2	11.2	5.6	56.1	3.90	7.1	8.35	46.4
Mexican American (F)	6.9	20.7	13.6	7.1	68.9	4.66	9.8	5.81	54.2
Black (M)	70.2	24.7	14.1	7.1	67.8	4.34	11.0	8.94	47.7
Black (F)	64.4	26.6	18.6	10.2	78.1	5.06	11.6	8.34	47.2
Anglo (M)	85.4	17.9	10.2	4.8	66.7	3.71	10.1	7.54	65.2
Anglo (F)	84.5	17.4	13.2	6.7	76.7	4.17	11.4	7.21	68.2
AGE 55-64									
Puerto Rican (M)	55.2	39.6	25.0	12.5	80.2	5.68	15.6	13.20	43.1
Puerto Rican (F)	51.7	46.7	31.7	16.7	80.8	7.15	13.3	10.19	45.2
Cuban (M)	84.1	18.3	9.5	4.8	65.1	5.00	9.5	10.00	48.4
Cuban (F)	73.2	26.9	12.1	7.4	77.2	4.71	15.4	9.96	61.5
Mexican American (M)	66.2	31.2	15.2	5.1	59.6	5.01	9.0	8.52	42.4
Mexican American (F)	58.9	33.1	20.2	10.6	71.6	5.46	10.6	7.39	45.0
Black (M)	59.1	37.2	18.2	8.9	72.5	5.15	14.5	9.34	42.6
Black (F)	54.9	39.7	22.0	10.8	79.4	5.68	11.9	8.77	41.1
Anglo (M)	75.8	30.4	12.8	5.5	72.6	4.35	13.7	8.27	58.3
Anglo (F)	76.4	26.8	14.1	6.6	77.0	4.55	12.1	7.91	59.9

AGE 65-74									
Puerto Rican (M)	66.0	49.1	18.9	11.3	83.0	5.93	13.2	9.71	48.5
Puerto Rican (F)	60.4	41.7	29.2	16.7	89.6	5.81	14.6	11.43	29.7
Cuban (M)	70.8	34.8	18.0	9.0	79.8	4.93	13.5	10.50	48.4
Cuban (F)	52.8	34.4	17.6	5.6	83.2	7.60	13.6	8.71	38.5
Mexican American (M)	58.6	44.9	20.1	12.8	73.1	4.91	17.1	9.40	35.3
Mexican American (F)	57.3	44.6	22.9	12.1	84.1	6.25	21.7	8.37	31.5
Black (M)	51.9	52.8	19.9	9.2	73.0	5.69	17.8	10.30	29.4
Black (F)	53.0	46.8	22.9	10.5	81.3	6.12	14.8	9.25	29.1
Anglo (M)	69.6	42.1	13.2	5.6	76.4	4.81	18.2	8.85	44.2
Anglo (F)	71.9	35.4	15.2	6.6	80.7	5.01	16.1	8.93	48.1
AGE 75-84									
Puerto Rican (M)	37.5	50.0	25.0	12.5	87.5	5.29	25.0	7.50	0.0
Puerto Rican (F)	25.0	81.3	37.5	31.3	93.8	7.87	43.8	8.43	0.0
Cuban (M)	67.6	43.2	16.2	8.1	86.5	6.03	24.3	6.78	27.3
Cuban (F)	69.7	39.4	9.1	3.0	87.9	6.41	12.1	7.75	36.8
Mexican American (M)	57.3	47.9	14.5	8.6	69.2	5.44	15.4	9.61	28.2
Mexican American (F)	51.4	57.5	28.1	14.4	86.3	6.34	21.9	8.47	19.8
Black (M)	53.3	56.0	18.3	9.9	72.9	5.74	20.5	10.11	18.2
Black (F)	51.2	53.9	24.7	11.1	82.6	6.24	18.4	9.79	21.9
Anglo (M)	67.4	49.0	14.8	6.8	79.6	5.10	22.6	9.28	34.0
Anglo (F)	69.4	44.0	17.2	7.5	82.8	5.40	20.2	9.03	36.5
AGE 85 and over									
Puerto Rican (M)	50.0	100.0	0.0	0.0	100.0	3.50	0.0	0.0	50.0
Puerto Rican (F)	77.8	55.6	0.0	0.0	66.7	5.67	22.3	15.0	16.7
Cuban (M)	100.0	0.0	0.0	0.0	0.0	0.0	0.0	0.0	0.0
Cuban (F)	66.7	83.3	0.0	0.0	91.7	6.09	16.7	9.50	10.0
Mexican American (M)	48.4	64.5	29.0	22.6	67.7	6.43	29.0	9.67	29.4
Mexican American (F)	54.1	75.7	32.4	21.6	75.7	5.36	21.6	8.00	11.8
Black (M)	48.1	67.9	20.8	13.2	69.8	5.66	19.8	11.81	12.7
Black (F)	53.4	70.8	22.8	12.3	77.6	5.92	18.7	10.54	10.4
Anglo (M)	68.5	59.3	14.2	8.5	79.3	5.06	25.2	9.42	24.9
Anglo (F)	68.3	62.2	18.2	10.0	80.5	5.19	22.7	9.22	22.9

*Taken from the pooled 1972, 1973, 1976, 1977, 1980, 1981, 1984, and 1985 Health Interview Surveys.

On the one hand, the objective (or medical-model–based) indicators are more accurate reflections of the physiological dimension of health status including signs, test results, and diagnosed disease entities. Conversely, the subjective (or functional-model–based) indicators are more accurate reflections of the individual's perception of and response to his or her physiological state. Thus, the objective indicators may be considered more accurate measures of the "need" for health care, whereas the subjective indicators may be considered more accurate measures of the "demand" for health care (Feldstein, 1983).

This distinction (need vs. demand) has important implications for studying the use of health services (Wolinsky, 1988). For example, if the health service under study is discretionary (e.g., initial visits to the doctor), then the subjective measures are more likely to have greater explanatory power. If, however, the health service under study is nondiscretionary (e.g., hospitalization rates), then the objective measures are more likely to have greater explanatory power. In circumstances in which the discretionary nature of the health service under study is somewhat mixed (e.g., rates for annual physician use), then both types of measures are likely to be predictive, but neither is likely to dominate. Thus, the selection of health status indicators can significantly alter the outcome of studies on the use of health services as well as the comparison of results across studies using different measures.

Mechanic (1979) has taken this issue a step further. In trying to reconcile the divergent findings of the two major schools of studies on the use of health services, Mechanic (1979) argues that:

> A major difficulty in surveys of health is the inadequacy of questionnaire indicators of illness and health status. Although questions on perceived health status, symptoms, chronic disease, and restricted activity are commonly asked, these usually reflect a complex pattern of illness perception and behavior that goes beyond the narrower conceptual definition of morbidity that researchers would, ideally, like to measure. (p. 390)

At the root of Mechanic's argument is the notion that subjective measures of health status represent the channeling of available data on the individual's physiological health state through his or her ontological being (i.e., what an individual defines to be his or her existence including what is both personally important and relevant). As a result, these subjective indicators (whether they be responses to questions about perceived health status, or self-reports of symptoms or conditions) are more measures of health behavior than they are of health status. That is why these measures are more predictive of use of health services than are other psychosocial or organizational factors.

Moreover, this pattern of findings suggests that the use of subjective (or functional) measures of health status, especially those obtained through social surveys, is inappropriate for establishing morbidity levels. Because one's ontological being derives from social processes, the rational calculus used to channel the available physiological data is relative to the individual's sociocultural and experiential heritage. As Mechanic (1979) notes, these underlying social processes account for why:

> persons with similar complaints behave so differently and why the same person with comparable symptoms at various times chooses to seek medical care on one occasion, but not on another. (p. 394).

These social processes also explain why some physiological signs or bodily changes become available data regarding one's health state (i.e., are perceived to exist by the individual, and are then recognized and classified as symptoms), and why some do not (Mechanic, 1980).

Another important issue is the way in which the use of health services is measured. Of particular interest is the unit of analysis employed (Andersen & Newman, 1973). Among the more frequently used are contact, volume, episode, and recency measures. Contact measures indicate whether or not a particular service was used during a defined catchment period. For example, Tables 2.1 and 2.2 contain measures of physician and hospital contact during the preceding year. These data indicate whether an individual saw a physician or spent a night in the hospital. Thus, contact measures focus more on access to the health service in question rather than on the amount of consumption. Accordingly, one would expect sociocultural and other background factors to exhibit their greatest impact on contact measures.

In contrast, volume measures indicate how many services were used during the catchment period. Typical examples (see Tables 2.1 and 2.2) include the number of physician visits or nights spent in the hospital during the preceding year. Thus, volume measures focus on consumption levels, implicitly assuming that some degree of access already existed. Accordingly, one would expect health status and the characteristics of the health care delivery system to exhibit their greatest impact on volume measures.

It would seem prudent, therefore, for any analysis of the use of health services to employ both contact and volume measures for each type of health behavior under study. The results should then be compared and contrasted to understand better individual level barriers to, and delivery system level catapults for, the use of health services (Wolinsky, 1988). In addition, because volume measures implicitly assume access exists, analysis of such measures should be restricted to those who have made contact (see Schur et al., 1987; Wolinsky, Coe, Mosely, & Homan, 1985). It is, after all, only logical to exclude nonusers from the analysis when the question is how much use occurred. The question of whether use occurred is addressed in the analysis of contact measures.

Episode measures take the notion of contact and volume one step forward by norming them to the emergence and sequelae of the illness event. That is, the catchment period becomes defined not in chronological time, but rather in terms of the illness episode. The advantage here is that more meaningful comparisons can be made because the use (whether in terms of contact or volume measures) is episode specific. For example, given the same illness episode, do different individuals have equal likelihood of contacting a physician? Among individuals with contact, does everyone have the same number of visits? The disadvantage lies in the increased complexities of data collection. Few individuals experience the same symptom episodes in any given catchment period, even though most experience some symptoms.

Recency measures of the use of health services are another matter. Frequently they take the form of asking the respondent how long it has been since they went to a physician. This involves several problems. One is that the categories seldom have equal intervals, with the two least recent categories typically being 5 or more years ago, and never. This makes the interpretation of product-moment–based analyses (e.g., regression) problematical, because it violates various underlying statistical assumptions (such as interval-level measurement, homoscedasticity, and multivariate normal distributions).

A second problem with recency measures involves the disjuncture between their catchment period and those of the independent variables that are used to predict them. The prediction of the use of health services that occurred 5 or more years ago, by current characteristics of the individual (especially factors like income, morale, living arrangements, and health status), defies logic unless one assumes that these characteristics are rather stable during reasonably long segments of the life course. That assumption appears untenable given the extant literature. (Note that to a much lesser extent the length of the catchment period can also be problematic for contact and volume measures, especially in terms of data aggregation and causal process issues [see Mechanic, 1979].)

Perhaps the most important problem with recency measures, however, is interpreting them. Although to some extent these measures capture an element of contact (access), a meaningful characterization of access can become rather obscured depending on the number and breadth of the catchment categories. There is no element of volume to them. Nor do they contain any element of an episode. Indeed, it is difficult to fathom exactly what the analysis of recency measures tells us about the use of health services. It would seem, therefore, that recency measures should not be used.

Modeling Issues

After the measures of health status and the use of health services have been selected, one is confronted with various options for modeling their analysis. Three related issues involved in making those selections warrant special attention. These are the differences between (a) categorical versus metric analyses, (b) limited versus saturated models, and (c) the functional forms of various predictive equation systems. In discussing the first, the traditional measure of perceived health status used in social survey research will serve as an example. Respondents in health surveys are typically asked how they would rate their health status; would they say it was excellent, good, fair, or poor?

To be sure, the perceived health status question elicits important information from the respondent. It initiates the process by which available data on the individual's physiological health state is channeled through his or her ontological being. Because the resulting definition of the situation has validity and meaning for the respondent, the only practical question is how that information is used by researchers in their statistical modeling. Most of the time the response categories are assigned numeric values ranging from 1 to 4, representing the metric (intervalized) coding procedures associated with regression analyses (see Branch et al., 1981; Evashwick et al., 1984; Wolinsky & Coe, 1984).

Does the metric coding of perceived health status optimally exploit the elicited information, however, or is it even legitimate? Both questions must be answered in the negative. The metric coding approach assumes that the difference between any two contiguous response categories is of equal importance for the outcome measure, such as physician use. It seems unlikely, for example, that the difference between reports of excellent versus good health has as much effect as the difference between reports of good versus fair health. The former captures more subtle differences between being in peak form versus not having any health problems, whereas the latter captures the recognition that something is not right with one's health. Unfortunately, the metric coding of the perceived health status question conceptually and statistically obscures these important distinctions. To capture these distinctions more fully (and maximize the effects of the categorical contrasts), the perceived health status measure should be dichotomized as excellent or good versus fair or poor (see Schur et al., 1987; for an excellent review of the construction, use, and power of dummy variables, see Polissar & Diehr, 1982). This issue also applies to various other categorical measures that are frequently treated as metric indices.

The second issue focuses on the use of limited versus saturated (i.e., fully specified, multivariate) analytic models. Having gone to some length to dispel the homogeneity assumption, and in the process noting the emergence of multivariate modeling focusing on the importance of the individual and his or her characteristics and traits, the call here for more saturated analytic models should come as no surprise. In addition to the logical demands that stem from the heterogeneity assumption, however, the assessment of the net or unique effects of each factor of interest requires more saturated (than limited) modeling.

Consider, for example, the case of assessing the net effects of widowhood on physician use and the contradictory evidence regarding this relationship. Consistent with the long-standing belief that widowhood has a profound (but perhaps not lasting) effect on the surviving spouse (Hyman, 1983), studies had (until recently) typically reported that widowed individuals go to a doctor and the hospital more often than married individuals (see Verbrugge, 1979). More recent work by Cafferata (1987) and Homan et al. (1986), however, reports that this is not the case.

The discrepancy between these two sets of studies is explained not so much by changes (which may or may not have occurred) in the effects of widowhood over time, but by changes in the way in which the use of health services has been modeled. Failing to control for living arrangements (i.e., whether the surviving spouse lived alone), the earlier studies attributed the observed differences in physician use to the effects of widowhood. In contrast, after controlling for living arrangements, the more recent studies found widowhood had no net effect. These studies attributed the observed differences in physician use to living alone.

The third modeling issue involves the functional form of the predictive equation system. Two points are to be considered here. These are the additivity and nonreciprocality assumptions of most modeling procedures (e.g., regression analysis). The additivity assumption holds that the effects of any particular factor (such as social supports) on the use of health services does not depend on the value of any other factor (such as gender or ethnicity). If it does, then regression analysis will result in biased estimates of the parameters of the analytic model, unless the appropriate statistical interaction terms are introduced, or the analyses are conducted separately within groups and the results compared across groups.

Unfortunately, good evidence exists, both conceptual and empirical, suggesting that the effects of many of the factors used to predict the use of health services differ for men and women (Verbrugge, 1985), and for whites and blacks (Keith & Ellis, 1987). Moreover, such statistical interaction is likely to occur when other outcomes are examined as well (Krause, 1988). Nonetheless, one seldom finds either the inclusion of the appropriate statistical interaction terms, or the comparison of separate analyses across groups (see Mutran & Ferraro, 1988). As a result, our confidence in the effects of one or another variable on the use of health services, as reported in the extant literature, must be somewhat discounted.

The other point about the functional form of predictive equation systems concerns the nonreciprocality assumption. In addition to assuming that no statistical interaction exists among the predictors, regression (and other) analyses assume that no reciprocal causation exists between any two or more factors in the model. If there is, it too leads to biased estimates of the model's parameters. Unfortunately, this problem is far more complex to resolve and requires the use of two-stage rather than ordinary least squares (OLS) regression techniques (see Heise, 1975).

Although the problematic reciprocal relationships may involve just independent variables (e.g., income and morale), both independent and dependent variables (e.g., morale and health status), or just dependent variables (e.g., physician and hospital use), the latter shall be underscored here. In particular, the failure to consider statistically the interplay between physician and hospital use would seem to be remarkable, especially given the consensus found in the conceptual literature about their relationship. As a result, little is known about how the consumption of one alters the potential for the use of the other (see Mutran & Ferraro, 1988). Given the increasing interest in substitution hypotheses (cf. Wolinsky et al. 1986), a continued aversion to nonreciprocal modeling techniques would seem ill advised.

Multiple Regression Analysis of HIS Data

A detailed, complex regression analysis that takes all of the preceding issues into simultaneous consideration is well beyond the scope of the present chapter. Indeed, it has regrettably not yet been attempted in the literature. Therefore, what is briefly presented next is the result of applying an additive, nonreciprocal, saturated model of health and the use of health services to the pooled HIS data. This is sufficient to demonstrate the basic importance of the conceptual and methodological issues described earlier for public policy concerning the health and health care of elderly Americans.

The standard multivariate approach that has been selected is Andersen's (1968) behavioral model of the use of health services. It has been frequently applied to the special case of the elderly (see Branch et al., 1981; Coulton & Frost, 1982; Evashwick et al., 1984; Eve, 1982, 1984; Eve & Friedsam, 1980; Mossey et al, 1988; Mutran & Ferraro, 1988; Stoller, 1982; Wan & Arling, 1983; Wan & Odell, 1981; Wolinsky & Coe, 1984; Wolinsky et al., 1983, 1988) and will be described in considerable detail in Chapter 3. Suffice it to say here that the behavioral model defines the use of health services as a function of the predisposing, enabling, and need characteristics of the *individual*. Predisposing characteristics reflect the fact that some individuals have a greater propensity to use health services than others, and that these propensities may be predicted by various characteristics before the onset of specific illness episodes. Typical indicators include age, marital status, living arrangements, race, education, and labor-force participation. Enabling characteristics reflect the fact that although some individuals may be predisposed to use health services, they will not unless they are able to do so. Typical indicators include family income, place of residence, and having a telephone (because in the HIS, telephone contacts with a physician are considered as visits). Need characteristics reflect the individual's perceived or evaluated health status, which is viewed as the basic and direct stimulus for use of health services given appropriate levels of the predisposing and enabling characteristics. Typical indicators include self-assessed health status and the extent of activity limitations owing to health conditions.

In the analyses reported in Table 2.3, the predisposing and enabling characteristics were coded as follows. Sex, widowhood, living arrangements, labor-force participation, place of residence, and possession of a telephone were coded as dummy variables (i.e., 0 or 1), with the presence of the trait described indexed as unity. Education was coded in the actual number of formal years attained, and income was coded in thousands of (1979 constant) dollars. A set of dummy variables was constructed to represent age, with the near-elderly (i.e., ages 45 to 64) as the reference (or omitted) category. Thus, the effects of each of the age dummy variables represent the difference between being in that age-group versus being near-elderly. A set of dummy variables was also constructed to represent ethnicity, with Anglos being the reference category.

A note on the dichotomous nature of several of the dependent variables is in order at this point. OLS regression techniques were used to estimate the parameters of the behavioral model, because extensive research has shown that when the split of a dichotomous dependent variable is within the 0.25/0.75 (and probably even the 0.10/0.90) range, OLS yields results comparable with logistic regression or discriminant function analyses when large samples are employed (see Cleary & Angel, 1984). In this rather large pooled sample, the splits are generally within these acceptable boundaries (the principal exception being bed disability days). Standard statistical techniques were used to assess the remaining assumptions of the OLS techniques (see Lewis-Beck, 1981).

Two important patterns are apparent in the results shown in Table 2.3. Both have considerable significance for public policy concerning the health and health behavior of elderly Americans. First, despite the large number of variables used in these predictive equations, little of the variance was explained (i.e., the R^2 levels range from .056 to .142). Although both better measurement of the independent and dependent variables, and more complex modeling techniques (as described earlier) might well result in moderate increments to the R^2 levels, most of the health and health behavior remains (and likely will remain) unexplained. This underscores the remarkable heterogeneity of the health of elderly Americans and their use of health services. Simply stated, if homogeneity existed within various subpopulations and sub-subpopulations, then the R^2 levels reported here would have been closer to unity than to 0. This is clearly not the case, however. Therefore, the continuation of a "risk factor approach" to health policy for the elderly is unlikely to prove effective.

The second important pattern in the results shown in Table 2.3 involves the effects of the predisposing, enabling, and need characteristics. Although the need characteristics are the most important predictors of use, three reasons exist why this should not be mistakenly construed as evidence for the equitable nature of the health care delivery system. First and foremost (and as indicated earlier), most of

Table 2.3 Unstandardized Regression Coefficients for Predisposing, Enabling, and Need Characteristics on the Health and Health Services Utilization Indicators*

	Limited activity	Perceived health	Physician contact	Hospital contact	Bed Disability days
PREDISPOSING					
Female	-.097[d]	.046[d]	.070[d]	-.011[d]	.012[d]
Widowed	.035[d]	.000	-.002	.006[a]	.003
Lives alone	-.025[d]	.061[d]	.029[d]	.007[b]	.006[b]
Education	-.011[d]	.019[d]	.006[d]	.000[a]	.000[d]
Employed	-.237[d]	.172[d]	-.004	-.024[d]	-.012[d]
Age 65-74	-.009[b]	.045[d]	.047[d]	.019[d]	-.022[d]
Age 75-84	.017[d]	.064[d]	.065[d]	.047[d]	-.022[d]
Age 85-94	.150[d]	.070[d]	.027[c]	.050[d]	-.011[b]
Age 94 or older	.253[d]	.142[d]	-.050	.045	-.010
Puerto Rican	.009	-.052[c]	.056[c]	.003	.059[d]
Cuban	-.094[d]	.059[d]	.021	-.016	-.000
Mexican	-.102[d]	.027[c]	-.037[d]	-.021[c]	.009[a]
Black	.017[d]	-.078[d]	.014[c]	-.026[d]	.009[d]
ENABLING					
Northeast	-.019[d]	.014[d]	.006	-.016[d]	.000
South	.025[d]	-.047[d]	.000	-.000	.002
West	.036[d]	.002	.005	-.020[d]	.007[c]
Lives on farm	-.004	-.008	-.024[d]	-.011[a]	-.018[d]
Lives in central city	-.000	-.003	-.001	-.004	.008[d]
Income	-.079[d]	.088[d]	.046[d]	.012[d]	-.000
Telephone	-.031[d]	.043[d]	.103[d]	.021[d]	-.016[d]
NEED					
Limited activity			.146[d]	.112[d]	.068[d]
Perceived health			-.091[d]	-.106[d]	-.086[d]
INTERCEPT	.714[d]	.264[d]	.494[d]	.158[d]	.117[d]
R²	.144	.135	.056	.068	.061
N	162,535	162,535	162,535	162,535	162,535

	Restricted activity days	Dental contact	Number of physician visits	Number of hospital nights	Number of hospital episodes
PREDISPOSING					
Female	.020[d]	.043[d]	.279[d]	-.405[d]	-.067[d]
Widowed	.005[d]	-.065[d]	.077[a]	.234[a]	.036[a]
Lives alone	.024[d]	.090[d]	.288[d]	.151	-.018
Education	.000	.030[d]	-.015[d]	-.012	.002
Employed	-.019[d]	.004	-.476[d]	-.803[d]	-.100[d]
Age 65-74	-.036[d]	-.058[d]	-.016	.436[d]	.016
Age 75-84	-.041[d]	-.115[d]	.043	.505[d]	-.024
Age 85-94	-.064[d]	-.194[d]	-.467[d]	.564[b]	-.032
Age 94 or older	-.077[b]	-.208[d]	-.351	.322	-.142
Puerto Rican	.060[d]	.039	.828[d]	.630	-.078
Cuban	-.014	.030	.712[d]	.443	.001
Mexican	-.000	.042[d]	.072	-.249	-.031
Black	.012[d]	-.038[d]	.312[d]	.301[b]	-.067[c]
ENABLING					
Northeast	-.000	.021[d]	.193[d]	.320[c]	-.043[b]
South	.004[a]	.013[c]	-.245[d]	-.295[c]	-.004
West	.025[d]	.037[d]	.227[d]	-1.107[d]	-.031
Lives on farm	-.022[d]	-.014	-.115[a]	-.381[a]	-.066[a]
Lives in central city	-.009[d]	.012[d]	.193[d]	.281[d]	-.044[c]
Income	-.002	.113[d]	.063[c]	.066	.005
Telephone	-.006	.096[d]	.256[d]	-.181	.007
NEED					
Limited activity	.165[d]	-.018[d]	1.945[d]	1.709[d]	.183[d]
Perceived health	-.149[d]	.035[d]	-1.879[d]	-1.413[d]	-.225[d]
INTERCEPT	.206[d]	-.075[d]	5.013[d]	8.718[d]	1.469[d]
R^2	.128	.160	.175	.113	.052
N	162,535	115,534	123,930	23,154	23,154

*Taken from the pooled 1972, 1973, 1976, 1977, 1980, 1981, 1984, and 1985 Health Interview Surveys.
[a] $p \leq .05$; [b] $p \leq .01$; [c] $p \leq .001$; [d] $p \leq .0001$.

the variance in the use of health services was unexplained. Thus, it is not yet at all certain why elderly Americans use or do not use health services. Second, although the direct effects of the predisposing and enabling characteristics on use are relatively modest, many of them are both statistically and substantively meaningful. These indicate the existence of both economic (e.g., income and employment status) and noneconomic (e.g., gender and ethnicity) barriers to access. Third, the predisposing and enabling characteristics explain about as much of the variance in the health status measures as they (i.e., the health status measures) do for the use measures. Thus, the predisposing and enabling factors also have indirect effects on use through their direct effects on health status. In sum, it would be erroneous to portray these results as indicative of equity in the health and health care of elderly Americans.

The effects of the dummy variables representing the age-groups also deserve special (but necessarily brief) mention here. Dental contact is the only outcome measure for which being in each successive age-group consistently has a significantly greater impact (i.e., poorer health or greater use). Elsewhere we have shown this exception to be a cohort and not an aging effect (Wolinsky & Arnold, 1989). For the remaining outcomes, the effects of age-group are varied, demonstrating both the inconsistency and limited utility of chronological age as a linear predictor of health and the use of health services. For example, those aged 65 to 74 and 85 to 94 are equally disadvantaged in terms of activity limitations relative to the near-elderly, whereas their 75- to 84-year-old counterparts are significantly less disadvantaged. Those aged 65 to 74 report significantly lower perceived health status than their near-elderly counterparts, whereas the older-elderly report significantly higher perceived health status. Among those who have seen a physician in the past year, only those aged 95 and older have significantly different volumes of use, and they see a physician less often. Among those who have been hospitalized in the past year, the near-elderly, the young-old, and the very-oldest-old all have comparable numbers of hospital episodes.

SUMMARY

This chapter has focused on what we do and do not know about the elderly's health and use of health services, with special attention paid to the heterogeneity issue. Four important points emerged from the preceding discussion. The first is that heterogeneity, indeed, exists in the health and health behavior of elderly Americans.

The second point is that health status has been consistently shown to be the single most important determinant of the use of health services, whether among the elderly population as a whole, among heavy users, or among low users. To be sure, the literature indicates that of the variance in health behavior that can be explained, most is accounted for by the direct effects of measures of health status (with chronological age contributing relatively little). This leads directly to the third point. Regardless of which predictive model is used or where the sample is drawn from, the amount of variance in the use of health services that can be explained is rather modest. Most applications of the behavioral model to the special case of elderly persons account for less than 25% of the variance in their use of health services.

It is the fourth point that is the most troubling, however. It involves the possibility that the measurement and modeling issues may play a significant role in the preceding two points. Regarding the dominance of the relationship between health status and the use of health services (second point), the subjective nature of functional health status measures makes them inappropriate for use in evaluating the equitable nature of the health care delivery system. They simply go too far beyond the conceptual domain of morbidity to be acceptable proxies in equity assessments. What has been demonstrated to date is that the consumption of health services is primarily a function of the demand for them. That is not isomorphic to demonstrating that the use of health services is primarily a function of need.

REFERENCES

Andersen, R. M. (1968). *A behavioral model of families' use of health services.* Chicago: Center for Health Administration Studies.

Andersen, R., Lewis, S., Giachello, A., Aday, L. A., & Chiu, G. (1981). Access to medical care among the Hispanic population of the southwestern United States. *Journal of Health and Social Behavior,22*, 78–89.

Andersen, R., & Newman, J. (1973). Societal and individual determinants of medical care utilization in the United States. *Milbank Memorial Fund Quarterly, 51*, 95–124.

Antonucci, T. C. (1985). Personal characteristics, social support, and social behavior. In R. H. Binstock & E. Shanas (Eds.), *Handbook of aging and the social sciences* (2nd ed.), (pp. 94–128). New York: Van Nostrand Reinhold.

Antonucci, T. C., & Akiyama, H. (1987). Social networks in adult life and a preliminary examination of the convoy model. *Journal of Gerontology, 42,* 519–527.

Berki, S., Lepowski, J., Wyszewianski, L., Landis, J. R., Magilavy, M. L., McLaughlin, C., & Murt, H. (1986). *High-volume and low-volume users of health services: United States, 1980.* (DHHS Publication No. 86-20402). Washington, D. C.: Government Printing Office.

Binstock, R. H. (1985). The oldest old: A frest perspective or compassionate ageism revisited. *Milbank Memorial Fund Quarterly, 63,* 420–451.

Bloom, B. S., & Soper, K. A. (1980). Health and medical care for the elderly and aged population: The state of the evidence. *Journal of the American Geriatrics Socity, 28,* 451–455.

Branch, L., Jette, A., Evashwick, C., Polansky, M., Rowe, G., & Diehr, P. (1981). Toward understanding elders' health service utilization. *Journal of Community Health, 7,* 80–92.

Butler, R. N. (1975). *Why survive? Being old in America.* New York: Harper & Row.

Cafferata, G. L. (1987). Marital status, living arrangements, and the use of health services by elderly persons. *Journal of Gerontology, 43,* 613–619.

Callahan, D. (1987). *Setting limits: Medical goals in an aging society.* New York: Simon & Schuster.

Cleary, P. D., & Angel, R. (1984). The analysis of relationships involving dichotomous dependent variables. *Journal of Health and Social Behavior, 25,* 334–348.

Cornoni-Huntley, J. C., Foley, D. J., White, L. R., Suzman, R., Berkman, L. F., Evans, D. A., & Wallace, R. B. (1985). Epidemiology of disability in the oldest old: Methodologic issues and preliminary findings. *Milbank Memorial Fund Quarterly, 63,* 350–376.

Coulton, C., & Frost, A. (1982). Use of social and health services by the elderly. *Journal of Health and Social Behavior, 23,* 330–339.

Department of Health and Human Services. (1988). *Health, United States, 1988* (DHHS Publication No. 88-1232). Washington, DC: Government Printing Office.

Evashwick, C., Rowe, G., Diehr, P., & Branch, L. (1984). Factors explaining the use of health care services by the elderly. *Health Services Research, 19,* 357–382.

Eve, S. B. (1982). Use of health maintenance organizations by older adults. *Research on Aging, 4,* 179–203.

Eve, S. B. (1984). Age strata differences in utilization of health care services among adults in the United States. *Sociological Focus, 17,* 105–120.

Eve, S. B., & Friedsam, H. (1980). Multivariate analysis of health care services utilization among older Texans. *Journal of Health and Human Resources Administration, 3,* 169–191.

Federal Council on Aging. (1981). *The need for long term care: Information and issues.* Washington, DC: Government Printing Office.

Feldstein, P. J. (1983). *Health care economics* (2nd ed.). New York: John Wiley & Sons.

Fuchs, V. (1974). *Who shall live? Health economics and social change.* New York: Basic Books.

Haug, M. R. (1981). Age and medical care utilization patterns. *Journal of Gerontology, 36,* 103–111.

Havlik, R. J., Liu, B. M., Kovar, M. G., Suzman, R., Feldman, J. J., Harris, T., & Van Nostrand, J. (1987). *Health statistics on older persons, 1986* (DHHS Publication No. 87-1409). Washington, DC: Government Printing Office.

Heise, D. (1975). *Causal analysis.* New York: John Wiley & Sons.

Homan, S. M., Haddock, C. C., Winner, C. A., Coe, R. M., & Wolinsky, F. D. (1986). Widowhood, sex, labor force participation, and the use of physician services by elderly adults. *Journal of Gerontology, 41*, 793–796.

Hyman, H. (1983). *Of time and widowhood*. Durham, NC: Duke University Press.

Jackson, J. J. (1967). Social gerontology and the Negro: A review. *The Gerontologist, 7*, 168–178.

Jackson, J. J. (1985). Race, national origin, ethnicity, and aging. In R. H. Binstock & E. Shanas (Eds.), *Handbook of aging and the social sciences* (2nd ed.), (pp. 264–303). New York: Van Nostrand Reinhold.

Kahn, R. L. (1979). Aging and social support. In M. Riley (Ed.), *Aging from birth to death* (pp. 77–91). Boulder, CO: Westview Press.

Kahn, R. L., & Antonucci, T. C. (1980). Convoys over the life course: Attachment, roles, and social support. In P. Baltes & O. Brim (Eds.), *Life-span development and behavior* (pp. 147–168). New York: Academic Press.

Keith, V. K., & Ellis, S. (1987, August). *Utilization of health services by the black and white elderly*. Paper presented at the annual meeting of the Society for the Study of Social Problems, Chicago, IL.

Kovar, M. G. (1977). Health of the elderly and use of health services. *Public Health Reports, 92*, 9–19.

Kovar, M. G. (1986). Expenditures for the medical care of elderly people living in the community in 1980. *The Milbank Quarterly, 64*, 100–132.

Krause, N. M. (1988). Social supports and well-being: Gender and ethnic differences. *Annual Review of Gerontology and Geriatrics, 8*, 171–192.

Lewis-Beck, M. S. (1981). *Applied regression*. Beverly Hills: Sage.

Lubitz, J., & Prihoda, R. (1983). Use and costs of Medicare services in the last years of life. In *Health, U.S., 1983* (DHHS Publication No. 84-1232). Washington, DC: Government Printing Office.

Mechanic, D. (1979). Correlates of physician utilization: Why do major multivariate studies of physician utilization find trivial psychosocial and organizational effects? *Journal of Health and Social Behavior, 20*, 387–396.

Mechanic, D. (1980). The experience and reporting of common physical complaints. *Journal of Health and Social Behavior, 21*, 146–155.

Mossey, J. M., Havens, B., & Wolinsky, F. D. (1988). The consistency of formal health care utilization. In M. Ory & K. Bond (Eds.), *Aging and the use of formal health services* (pp. 81–98). New York: Tavistock Publications.

Mossey, J. M., & Roos, L. L. (1987). Using claims to measure health status: The illness scale. *Journal of Chronic Diseases, 40*, 71–78.

Mossey, J. M., & Shapiro, E. (1985). Physician use by the elderly over an eight-year period. *American Journal of Public Health, 75*, 1333–1334.

Mutran, E., & Ferraro, K. J. (1988). Medical need and use of health services among older adults: Examination of gender and racial differences. *Journal of Gerontology, 43*, S162–S171.

Neugarten, B. L. (1974). Age groups in American society and the rise of the young old. *Annals of the American Academy of Political and Social Science, 415*, 187–198.

Neugarten, B. L. (1979). Age or need entitlement. In J. Hubbard (Ed.), *Aging: Agenda for the eighties* (pp. 48–52). Washington, DC: Government Research Corporation.

Neugarten, B. L. (1982). Policy for the 1980s: Age or need entitlement? In B. L. Neugarten (Ed.), *Age or need?* (pp. 19–32). Beverly Hills: Sage Publications.

Polissar, L., & Diehr, P. K. (1982). Regression analysis in health services research: The use of dummy variables. *Medical Care*, 20, 959–974.

Report of the Secretary's Task Force on Black and Minority Health. (1985). Washington, DC: Government Printing Office.

Roos, N. P., Montgomery, P., & Roos, L. L. (1987). Health care utilization in the years prior to death. *The Milbank Quarterly*, 65, 231–254.

Russell, L. (1981). An aging population and the use of medical care. *Medical Care*, 19, 633–643.

Saenz, R., & Aguirre, B. E. (1988). *Mexican descent and ethnic self-conception*. Unpublished manuscript. Department of Sociology, Texas A&M University, College Station, Texas.

Schur, C. L., Bernstein, A. B., & Berk, M. L. (1987). The importance of distinguishing Hispanic subpopulations in the use of medical care. *Medical Care*, 25, 627–641.

Shanas, E., & Maddox, G. L. (1985). Health, health resources, and the utilization of care. In R. H. Binstock & E. Shanas (Eds.), *Handbook of aging and the social sciences* (2nd ed.), (pp. 697–726). New York: Van Nostrand Reinhold.

Snider, E. L. (1981). Young-old versus old-old and the use of health services: Does the difference make a difference? *Journal of the American Geriatrics Society*, 29, 354–358.

Soldo, B. J., & Manton, K. G. (1985). Changes in the health status and service needs of the oldest old: Current patterns and future trends. *Milbank Memorial Fund Quarterly*, 63, 286–323.

Stoller, E. P. (1982). Patterns of physician utilization by the elderly: A multivariate analysis. *Medical Care*, 20, 1080–1089.

Suzman, R., & Riley, M. W. (1985). Introducing the "oldest old." *Milbank Memorial Fund Quarterly*, 63, 177–186.

Suzman, R., & Willis, D. (Eds.). (1988). *The oldest old*. New York: Oxford University Press.

Travino, F. M., & Moss, A. J. (1984). *Health indicators for Hispanic, black, and white Americans* (DHHS Publication No. 84-1576). Washington, DC: Government Printing Office.

Verbrugge, L. M. (1979). Marital status and health. *Journal of Marriage and the Family*, 41, 267–285.

Verbrugge, L. M. (1985). Gender and health: An update on hypotheses and evidence. *Journal of Health and Social Behavior*, 26, 157–177.

Wan, T. T. H., & Arling, G. (1983). Differential use of health services among disabled elderly. *Research on Aging*, 5, 411–431.

Wan, T. T. H., & Odell, B. G. (1981). Factors affecting the use of social and health services among the elderly. *Ageing and Society*, 1, 95–115.

Wolinsky, F. D. (1988). *The sociology of health: Principles, practitioners, and issues* (2nd ed.). Belmont, CA: Wadsworth Publishing.

Wolinsky, F. D., & Arnold, C. L. (1988). A different perspective on health and health services utilization. *Annual Review of Gerontology and Geriatrics*, 8, 71–101.

Wolinsky, F. D., & Arnold, C. L. (1989). A birth cohort analysis of dental contact among elderly Americans. *American Journal of Public Health*, 79, 47–51.

Wolinsky, F. D., Arnold, C. L., & Nallapati, I. V. (1988). Explaining the declining rate of physician utilization among the oldest-old. *Medical Care*, 26, 544–553.

Wolinsky, F. D., & Coe, R. M. (1984). Physician and hospital utilization among noninstitutionalized elderly adults: An analysis of the Health Interview Survey. *Journal of Gerontology, 39,* 334–341.

Wolinsky, F. D., Coe, R. M., Miller, D. K., Prendergast, J. M., Creel, M. J., & Chavez, M. N. (1983). Health services utilization among the noninstitutionalized elderly. *Journal of Health and Social Behavior, 24,* 325–337.

Wolinsky, F. D., Coe, R. M., Mosely, R. R., & Homan, S. M. (1985). Veterans' and nonveterans' use of health services: A comparative analysis. *Medical Care, 24,* 1358–1371.

Wolinsky, F. D., Mosely, R. R., & Coe, R. M. (1986). A cohort analysis of the use of health services by elderly Americans. *Journal of Health and Social Behavior, 27,* 209–219.

Chapter 3

Design and Method

The purpose of this chapter is to present the reader with the overall design of the study. As such, it serves as the conceptual and empirical foundation for the remainder of the book. To do this, the present chapter is divided into four major sections. The first details the selection of the design matrix that drives the study. This includes both a theoretical and methodological justification of the eight-cohort-by-four-survey design, and an overview of the Health Interview Surveys (HISs) from which the data are taken. The second section of the chapter describes the behavioral model of the use of health services that provides the conceptual framework for the regression-based cohort analysis. Included in this section is an overview of the intellectual development and modification of the behavioral model, as well as its particular relevance for and application to the special case of the elderly.

The regression-based cohort analytic techniques developed specifically for use in this study are described in the third section of the chapter. Two new approaches are presented. The first provides estimates of the age, period, and cohort effects net of the other characteristics identified in the behavioral model, and the second facilitates the assessment of whether these other characteristics are themselves affected by age, period, or cohort effects. The final section of the chapter presents the coding algorithms, means, and standard deviations of the indicators used to operationalize the predisposing, enabling, and need characteristics, as well as the measures of the use of health services specified in the behavioral model.

SELECTION OF COHORTS AND DATA

The objective of this study is to allow the age-stratification perspective (discussed in Chapter 1) to inform a cohort analysis (the traditional components of which were also discussed in Chapter 1) of the health and health behavior of elderly Americans. This poses two immediate concerns. The first is that an overall design must be selected that provides an appropriate opportunity to assess the effects of age, period, and cohort. The second is that data must be obtained that are up to the analytical tasks at hand. Although these issues are intertwined, they shall be addressed separately.

Eight-Cohort-by-Four-Survey Design

Data on approximately 125,000 elderly individuals were pooled from the 1972, 1973, 1976, 1977, 1980, 1981, 1984, and 1985 Health Interview Surveys (which are described later). Eight 4-year cohorts were selected. Members of the youngest cohort (i.e., cohort 1) were 56 to 59 years old in 1972. Members of the oldest cohort (i.e., cohort 8) were 96 to 99 years old in 1984. To illustrate the design of the study, Table 3.1 shows the age composition, cohort designation, and number of cases per cohort in the four pooled survey-sets.

Using these particular cohorts has considerable theoretical advantages for detecting aging, period, and cohort effects. In terms of aging effects, each of these eight cohorts moves through several meaningful life-cycle stages during the 12 years in which they can be followed. For example, consider the youngest of the cohorts. Cohort 1 enters the table in the preretirement years (i.e., their late 50s). In addition to beginning to prepare for that transition, the members of this cohort are also faced with rendering assistance to their surviving elderly parents (usually their mothers) whose median age is 85 (see Torrey, 1985). By the time the members of cohort 1 leave the table, they are in their early 70s, have retired, have most likely lost their parents, and now have children of their own who have reached their 50s. Thus, the members of cohort 1 will have experienced a considerable shift in their position in the intergenerational transfer pattern (see Bengston, Cutler, Mangen, & Marshall, 1985; Rosow, 1985).

Consider the oldest of the cohorts. When cohort 8 enters the table, its members are just reaching their mid-80s. As such the average age of their children is about 59 years (see Torrey, 1985). As indicated in Chapter 1, this should facilitate the opportunity for the members of cohort 8 to receive more informal support (and possibly to substitute

Table 3.1 Age Composition, Cohort Designation (in Parentheses), and Number of Cases Per Cohort in Four Pooled Survey-Sets*

Age-group	Survey year			
	1972-73	1976-77	1980-81	1984-85
56-59	9,839 (1)	8,910 (9)	8,684 (9)	7,671 (9)
60-63	8,739 (2)	8,056 (1)	7,883 (9)	7,228 (9)
64-67	7,560 (3)	6,999 (2)	6,871 (1)	6,416 (9)
68-71	6,158 4)	5,843 (3)	5,680 (2)	5,596 (1)
72-75	4,757 (5)	4,492 (4)	4,337 (3)	4,344 (2)
76-79	3,479 (6)	3,219 (5)	3,030 (4)	3,302 (3)
80-83	2,137 (7)	2,100 (6)	1,986 (5)	1,988 (4)
84-87	1,030 (8)	1,049 (7)	1,117 (6)	1,158 (5)
88-91	430 (9)	416 (8)	425 (7)	514 (6)
92-95	128 (9)	121 (9)	126 (8)	142 (7)
96-99	33 (9)	31 (9)	46 (9)	38 (8)
Totals	44,290	41,236	40,1853	8,397

*For simplicity, cohorts that enter or leave the table are designated as cohort 9.

it for the use of formal health services [see Brody, 1985; Wolinsky, Mosely, & Coe, 1986) from their children. But by the time that this cohort leaves the table, its surviving members will have reached their late 90s. At that point they more than likely will experience a shift in the intergenerational transfer pattern inasmuch as their children will by then be entering their mid-70s. Thus, important age-strata comparisons in the use of health services can be made by using data on the youngest and oldest cohorts, as well as those that lie between them.

The relevance of the opportunities for detecting cohort effects can also be seen by comparing the life-cycle stages of the youngest and oldest cohorts at three important points during the 20th century (viz., World War I, the Great Depression, and World War II). Members of the youngest cohort were preschoolers during World War I, adolescents during the Great Depression, and young adults during World War II. In contrast, members of the oldest cohort were young adults (likely with their own families) during World War I, adults (with their children searching for a way to enter the labor force themselves) during the Great Depression, and middle aged (likely with their children serving in the armed forces while they cared for the grandchildren) during World War II.

Thus, although all eight cohorts lived through these same important times, they did so at different stages in the life cycle. As a result, it is reasonable to expect that they have been differentially affected by these historical events (see Elder, 1974, 1975). This may result in different patterns of the use of health services utilization by cohort. Older cohorts may use fewer services (especially through governmental programs like Medicare) because of their aversion to accepting, or relying on, external supports. In contrast, younger cohorts may be more likely to have been socialized to the view that they are entitled to such programs (see Binstock, 1985; Butler, 1975).

Finally, although these data cover only the period from 1972 to 1985, it was precisely during this time that remarkable changes in the financing of health care for the elderly occurred. For example, the implementation of Medicare and Medicaid in 1965 started an upward spiral on the use of health services by elderly Americans (see Anderson, 1985). To compensate for the rapid increases observed by 1977, the federal government began to introduce various cost-containment measures. Although several intermediary steps occurred along the way, the most notable of these was the shift from the fee-for-service system to the use of Diagnostic Related Groups (DRGs) as the method of payment under the Prospective Payment System (PPS). Introduced in 1983 as part of the Tax Equity and Fiscal Responsibility Act, DRGs have had a significant effect in reducing the length of hospital stays (see Wolinsky, 1988).

As a result of these changes in health care financing, it is reasonable to anticipate period effects in the elderly's use of health services. Building on the work of Aday, Andersen, and Fleming (1980) and Aday, Fleming, and Andersen (1984), the inverted curvilinear (Ushaped) pattern might look something like this. Between 1972 and 1976 the use of health services should have increased substantially given the enhanced access brought about by the Medicare and Medicaid programs. By 1980 these gains should have come to a halt, if not begun to erode. By 1984 the dramatic impacts of DRGs should have steepened the downward trajectory of the elderly's rates of health services use.

HISs

As indicated earlier, HISs have been selected as the source of data for this study. The HIS is an ongoing annual survey that first began in 1956 as authorized by Public Law 84-652. To this day, the HIS remains as the principal source of all "official" statistics on the health and use of health services in the United States. Because it is such a well-known data source, it will only be briefly described here. A more detailed description of the history, design, and logistics of the HISs can be found in several publications of the National Center for Health Statistics (see Department of Health and Human Services, 1975, 1985), under whose control it falls.

Basically, the HIS follows a multistage probability design that permits a continuous sampling of the noninstitutionalized civilian population of the United States. The sampling design is such that each week a representative sample of the United States population is interviewed. In the first stage of the weekly sampling process about 400 primary sampling units (PSUs) are randomly selected from the Census Bureau's universe of some 2,000 such geographically defined units. Collectively, these PSUs cover the 50 states and the District of Columbia. After a series of successive sampling steps, final sampling units (i.e., segments) are selected. Segments are defined to include four adjacent households.

Within each selected household, all competent and available members of the household are personally interviewed. Repeated call-backs are used to obtain interviews with competent adults who were not available at the time of the original interview. When such repeated call-backs are unsuccessful, or in the case of children or incompetent adults, the desired information is obtained from the most knowledgeable adult proxy available. Elsewhere it has been shown that the reliance on this proxy reporting system poses no substantive or policy limitations for modeling the use of health services among adults in the HISs (see Mosely & Wolinsky, 1986).

In summary, then, the HISs multistage sampling process results in 52 weekly replicated samples. These are pooled at the end of the calendar year, providing data on the approximately 110,000 individuals who reside in the 42,000 selected households. This pooled sample is fully representative of all individuals from all places during all seasons. It is, therefore, unnecessary to adjust the pooled data for seasonal and geographical fluctuations.

Notice that the smallest cell entries in Table 3.1 (i.e., those with fewer than 100 cases) all occur for the very oldest age-group (i.e., those older than age 95). This is as expected, inasmuch as the HISs are proportionately stratified by age, sex, and color (i.e., race) to ensure that they are representative of the United States population as a whole. All of the other cells in Table 3.1 contain more than a sufficient number of cases for analytic purposes (see Glenn, 1977). Indeed, the average size of the cells is approximately 5,000 cases, and it is only those age-groups older than age 87 for which fewer than 1,000 cases per cell exist. In general, this serves to minimize (if not eliminate) the sampling variation problems described in Chapter 1. Nonetheless, discussions of aging, period, or cohort effects detected among the nonagenarians will proceed with caution.

BEHAVIORAL MODEL OF
THE USE OF HEALTH SERVICES

As indicated in Chapter 2, many factors in addition to age influence the health status and use of health services by elderly Americans. Almost as many approaches exist to modeling them (see McKinlay, 1972, 1985; Wan, 1988; Ward, 1977; Wolinsky, Coe, & Mosely, 1987). The most widely used approach, however, is the behavioral model of the use of health services developed by Andersen (1968), and subsequently revised with various colleagues (see Andersen & Newman, 1973; Aday & Andersen, 1974, 1975; Aday et al., 1980, 1984).

Several reasons exist why this model has become and remained so popular (see Wan, 1988; Wolinsky, 1988). First, it is rather eclectic in its approach, combining a diversity of discipline-oriented perspectives. Second, it permits an assessment of the equity in the distribution of the use of health and health services that has considerable import for policy making. Third, it can be rather straightforwardly applied to survey data routinely collected by agencies of the federal government, such as the HISs. Fourth, it has considerable intuitive appeal. For these reasons the behavioral model of the use of health services has been selected as the conceptual framework that guides the cohort analysis outlined earlier.

Original Model

The original publication of the behavioral model of the use of health services appeared in 1968. It was a revision of Andersen's doctoral dissertation of the same year in sociology at Purdue University. As in all discipline-based dissertations, Andersen felt a need to establish early the theoretical importance of studying the use of health services. His justification of its sociological relevance bears repeating here (1968):

> Theoretically, use of health services can be viewed simply as another form of human behavior. Consequently, the sociologist can study utilization using the same theory and methods he might employ to study voting behavior or work role behavior. It might be argued that health and illness behavior are unique among the various types of social behavior because of the importance of the seemingly "non-social" variables of biology and disease. However, Zola [1964, p. 17] points out that, "It is not merely that there are social and psychological factors in illness but that illness is a social and psychological phenomenon. It cannot be understood or have any meaning without reference to a social context." (p. 3)

It was the purpose of Andersen's behavioral model to place the use of health services within such a context.

Practical reasons also existed for studying the use of health services. Andersen (1968) described what was then seen as a most urgent social problem as follows:

> The practical relevance of utilization studies stems, in large part, from their contribution to our understanding of the problems of distributing health services. The social significance of these problems grows with increasing societal support for the idea that access to medical care is a right of all men regardless of their personal resources. Yet, in actuality, considerable differences remain among various segments of the population with respect to the type and quantity of health services they use. The problems of distribution are magnified by rising expenditures for medical care. These increasing expenditures represent a significant shift in the allocation of resources in this country. Since World War II expenditures for health

have risen from less than four per cent to over six per cent of the gross national product. In absolute amount, expenditures are approaching 50 billion dollars a year. (pp. 3–4)

As ominous as the practical implications of the access to and financing of health care may have seemed then, the problem pales by comparison to that of today. Nearly 12% of the gross national product or $300 billion was spent on health care during 1987, causing some to suggest that limits be placed on the public's obligation to provide health care for the elderly under the Medicare and Medicaid programs (see Callahan, 1987).

Andersen (1968) chose the family as his unit of analysis. His argument was that the family:

has generally been considered an appropriate unit for studying consumption patterns of most consumer goods and services because it is the primary earning, spending, and consuming unit in our society. The family seems particularly appropriate for analyses of health service utilization because of changing needs for medical care through the family life cycle and because the family as a unit often decides what medical care a family member will receive. (p. 5)

Thus, Andersen (1968) anticipated a strong linkage between family life-cycle stage and health care decision making. Note that his reference to the life-cycle stage of the family is consonant with the life-course perspective that subsequently came to dominate sociological studies of the aging process (see Hagestad & Neugarten, 1985; Maddox, 1979).

Building on the earlier work of Anderson (1963), Andersen (1968) set out to integrate the then two major approaches to modeling health services use. On the one hand, the analyses of Feldstein (1964), Rosenthal (1964), Wirick (1966), and Theodore (1966) had focused on the tastes and preferences of consumers during the initial stages of an illness episode. Their focus switched to more economic factors such as income, insurance coverage, price, and access at the point of consumption. Conversely, the analyses of Rosenstock (1966), Stoeckle, Zola, and Davidson (1963), and Suchman (1965) focused more on social-psychological factors. These included the perceived severity of and susceptibility to illness, the relative ratio of the cost of seeking care to its beneficial effects, and those social structural factors that lead members of different reference groups to have either favorable or unfavorable attitudes toward scientific medicine.

Andersen (1968) thought that each approach had important elements, and that these must be incorporated into a more comprehensive model. Therefore, he borrowed heavily from these studies, specifically placing an emphasis on the family as the unit of analysis, separating the social-psychological factors from the economic ones, disaggregating the different types of health services from each other, incorporating perceptions of health and illness, and specifying the causal nexus of the preceding for the use of health services. The result was the three-stage model shown in Figure 3.1. In this model, the use of health services is seen as a sequential and conditional function of the family's predisposition to use health services, their ability to obtain them, and their need to consume them. Hence, the causal arrows flow from left to right.

The predisposing component in the model reflects the fact that some families have a greater propensity to use health services than others. Such propensities can be predicted before the onset of a specific illness episode based on current family characteristics. Families with these characteristics are more likely to use health services than those without them. As indicated in Figure 3.1, the predisposing component of the model is further subdivided into three dimensions including family composition, social structure, and health beliefs. The conceptual underpinnings of this component are directly linked to the Durkheimian perspective (see Durkheim, 1933, 1951), from which much of the logic and methods of social epidemiology are said to have emerged (see Ibrahim, 1983; Mechanic, 1978; Paul, 1966).

In the original application of the behavioral model, the family composition dimension was measured by the age, sex, and marital

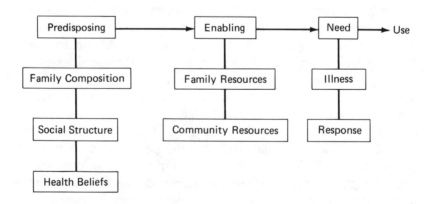

Figure 3.1 Behavioral model of use of health services.

Source: From Andersen, R. M. (1968). *A behavioral model of families' use of health services.* Chicago: Center for Health Administration Studies. Reprinted by permission.

status of the head of the family, family size, and the age of the oldest
and youngest family members. These indicators were thought to tap
the family's relative life-cycle position. The social structural dimension was measured by the main breadwinner's employment, social
class standing, occupation, education, race, and ethnicity. These characteristics were thought to tap the family's location in the social
structure and the behavioral patterns (i.e., life-styles) to which individuals in such positions became socialized. In addition, these characteristics are also thought to influence one's life chances. The health
beliefs dimension was measured by a series of questions about attitudes toward medical care, physicians, and disease. It was assumed
(Andersen, 1968) that "what a family thinks about health may ultimately influence health and illness behavior" (p. 16). When taken
together, the three dimensions of the predisposing component represent the social-psychological aspect of the behavioral model.

The enabling component reflects the fact that although the family
may be predisposed to use health services, it must nonetheless have
some means for obtaining them. It is the enabling component, then,
that contains those factors that make health services available to the
family for consumption. As indicated in Figure 3.1, Andersen (1968)
further subdivided this component into two dimensions. The first
consists of the family's resources. In the original study this dimension
was measured by family income, savings, the presence of health
insurance, having a regular source of care, and being on welfare. These
measures were thought to tap the family's ability to provide for itself.
The second dimension consists of the community's resources. They
are important because a family's ability to pay for health care is
relevant only if appropriate services can be conveniently purchased.
The original indicators of community resources were physician- and
hospital-bed-to-population ratios, as well as the geographical location
and population density of the place of residence. When taken together, the two dimensions of the enabling component represent the
economic aspect of the behavioral model.

Although the predisposing and enabling components are necessary
conditions for the use of health services, they are not sufficient ones.
To use health services, the family must perceive some illness (or its
possibility) among its members. This need is the "most immediate
cause of health service use" (Andersen, 1968, p. 17). As indicated in
Figure 3.1, need is further subdivided into two dimensions. The first
represents the amount of illness that is perceived by the family to
exist. It was originally measured by perceived health status, the
number of symptoms reported, the number of disability days taken,

and the amount of "free care" obtained. These indicators tap the family's recognition that a health problem either exists or is on the horizon. The second dimension represents the patterned reaction of the family to the perception of illness. It was originally measured by an indicator of whether members of the family usually see a physician when symptoms are recognized, and whether regular physician check-ups are scheduled. These indicators tap the family's routine behavioral response to health threats and their emphasis on health maintenance. When taken together, the two dimensions of the need component represent the preventive and health behavior component of the model.

The last component of the behavioral model is the outcome of primary interest, the use of health services. Although not shown in Figure 3.1, Andersen (1968) identified two types of use behavior in which families engage. These are discretionary and nondiscretionary behavior. The former represents those health services whose use is primarily a function of family choice. In contrast, the latter represents those health services whose use is primarily a function of the health care provider. An example of discretionary use involves going to see the dentist. Such decisions are most likely to be a function of the family's values and available income. In contrast, whether a family member is hospitalized is most likely to be a decision made by the physician, acting as a fiduciary agent for the individual and his or her family (see Parsons, 1951, 1958, 1975). Physician use falls somewhere in the middle, because initial visits for an illness episode will likely be a function of perceived need (a decision made by the family), whereas follow-up visits will likely be a function of the practice pattern of the provider (i.e., a decision made by the physician).

Although they did not specifically label the issue as discretionary versus nondiscretionary use, Anderson and Sheatsley (1967) had earlier made this point quite well:

> The patient exercises judgement and discretion whether or not to seek physician services. . . . Once the patient has sought physician services, the patient's judgement and discretion are greatly reduced and the patient begins to follow the physician's judgement and discretion. The clear impression . . . is that patients overwhelmingly tend to follow physicians' recommendations regarding hospital related physicians' services as reported by both patients and physicians. (p. 84)

Thus, one would expect that the salience of the components shown in Figure 3.1 would be greatest at the left end of the process for discretionary use, and greatest at the right end of the process for nondiscretionary use.

In summary, Andersen's (1968) conceptualization of families' use of health services can be consolidated into the three formal hypotheses:

> *Hypothesis I.* The amount of health services used by a family will be a function of the predisposing and enabling characteristics of the family and its need for medical care. Each of the three components will make an independent contribution to the understanding of differences in use of health services. *Hypothesis II.* The explanatory components of the model will vary in their contribution to the explanation of total use. Need will be more important than the predisposing and enabling components because it represents factors most directly related to use. *Hypothesis III.* The contribution of each component will vary according to the type of health service: (1) the contribution of need will be greatest for hospital services because these are defined as most necessary and the family has the least discretion in choosing alternative actions; (2) the contribution of the predisposing and enabling components will be greatest for dental services because these are defined as least necessary and the family has the most discretion in choosing alternative actions; (3) all of the components will contribute to understanding physician utilization because they are defined as less necessary than hospital services but more necessary than dental services. (pp. 19–20)

Using data on the 2,367 families surveyed as part of the 1963 nationwide household study of the University of Chicago's Center for Health Administration Studies, Andersen found considerable support for his model. Overall, he was able to explain 27% of the variation in families' hospital use, 47% of the variation in their physician use, and 19% of the variation in their dental use.

Nonetheless, Andersen (1968) was forced to modify his model somewhat. Figure 3.2 shows the original model (panel A), the modified model for hospital use (panel B), the supported model for physician use (panel C), and the modified model for dental use (panel D). With the exception of young families' predisposition to use obstetrical services, the predisposing and enabling characteristics were relatively unrelated to the use of hospitals. The main predictor here was the need component. In contrast, the use of physician services was consistent with the original model. The use of dental services was also relatively consistent with the original model, inasmuch as the predisposing and enabling components were salient, although the measures of medical need were rather unimportant.

A. The Hypothesized Sequence

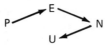

B. The Observed Model for Hospital Use

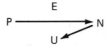

C. The Observed Model for Physician Use

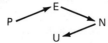

D. The Observed Model for Dental Use

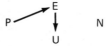

Figure 3.2 Causal relationships among predisposing, enabling, and need components, and use of health services.
Source: Adapted from Andersen, R. M. (1968). *A behavioral model of families' use of health services*. Chicago: Center for Health Administration Studies. Reprinted by permission.

Subsequent Modifications of Behavioral Model

Although the preceding discussion has indicated that the initial application of the behavioral model was rather successful, it was soon modified by Andersen and colleagues (see Aday & Andersen, 1974, 1975; Andersen & Newman, 1973). Two major changes warrant particular attention here. The first change involves a shift, at least directly, from the family as the unit of analysis to the individual as the unit of analysis. In the original model, the use of health services by all family members was combined into summary indices based on the California Relative Value Scale (California Medical Association, 1960). That scale assigned work-unit equivalents to all types of hospital, physician, and dental services. These were then summed across family members.

There were problems then, just as there are now, with the construction of relative value scales (see Hsiao, 1988). More important, however, was the problem of interpreting such a measure that had been aggregated across all family members. Although two families with combined relative value totals of 300 each had indeed used equivalent amounts of services in the aggregate, the patterns nested within that use could be quite different. For example, what if one family's use was equally distributed across all of its family members, whereas the other family's use all resulted from the father's acute myocardial infarction? Would not an assessment using the individual rather than the family as the unit of analysis provide for a different interpretation? It most certainly would. Thus, although the family remained (at least implicitly) the unit of analysis at the conceptual level, the use of health services was disaggregated to focus on each individual member of the family (see Andersen & Newman, 1973). Among other points, this also facilitated a more precise assessment of the relative equity in the use of health services between various target groups, such as children and the elderly.

The second major change in the behavioral model was its emphasis on more than just the characteristics of the individual. As Andersen and Newman (1973) note:

> The utilization of health services can be viewed as a type of individ-
> ual behavior. In general the behavioral sciences have attempted to
> explain individual behavior as a function of characteristics of the
> individual himself, characteristics of the environment in which he
> lives, and/or some interaction of these individual and societal forces
> (Moore, 1969). To date, most of the empirical studies and theories
> dealing with health services utilization have emphasized the individ-
> ual characteristics while less attention has been paid to the societal
> impact. (p. 96)

Accordingly, they set about outlining a framework that more explicitly took both the individual and societal factors into account.

Figure 3.3 shows the relationships of the societal and individual factors with each other, with the health services system, and with the use of health services. Andersen and Newman (1973) thought that the main societal forces at work were medical technology and social norms. The major components of the health services system were the volume and distribution of resources, and their organization in terms of access and structure. As indicated in Figure 3.3, the societal characteristics affect the individual directly, as well as indirectly through their impact on the health services system. Thus, their impact on the use of health services was only indirect. In contrast, the characteristics of the individual are the direct causes of the use of health services.

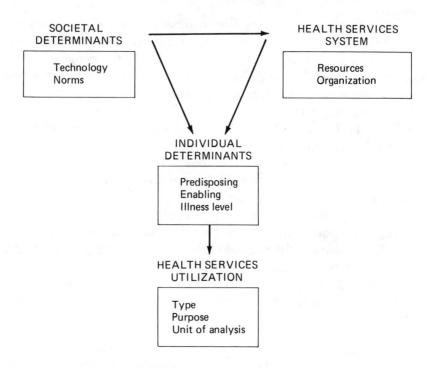

Figure 3.3 Addition of societal determinants and health services system to behavioral model.

Source: Andersen, R. M. & Newman, J. F. (1973). Societal and individual determinants of medical care utilization in the United States. *Milbank Memorial Fund Quarterly, 51*, 95–124. Reprinted by permission.

Ultimately, these modifications really only represent a modest revision of the behavioral model of the use of health services. After summarizing them, Andersen and Newman (1973, p. 107) graphically portrayed the model as shown in Figure 3.4. A careful examination of it reveals only four major changes from the original (see Figure 3.1). First, the use of health services and the arrow leading to it from the need component have been omitted for clarity. Second, the family composition dimension of the predisposing component has been relabeled as the demographic dimension, in keeping with the shift to the individual as the explicit unit of analysis. Third, the need component has been relabeled as the illness level, and its two dimensions have been relabeled as perceived (by the individual) and evaluated (by a health professional). Fourth, more indicators are listed as tapping each component and its various dimensions.

Using data from three sources (Andersen, 1968; Andersen, Smedby, & Anderson, 1970; Newman, 1971), Andersen and Newman (1973) were able to demonstrate considerable support for the revised model. This is summarized in Table 3.2, which indicates the relative importance of the dimensions of each of the three components of the model in predicting the use of hospital, physician, and dentist services. Again, these results are rather consistent with those reported in the original assessment of the model.

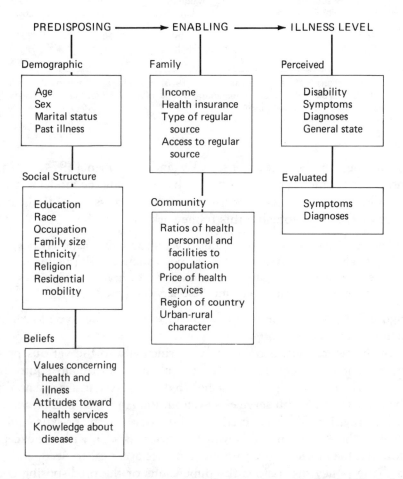

Figure 3.4 Graphic portrayal of revised version of behavioral model.
Source: Andersen, R. M. & Newman, J. F. (1973). Societal and individual determinants of medical care utilization in the United States. *Milbank Memorial Fund Quarterly, 51,* 95–124. Reprinted by permission.

Table 3.2 Relative Importance of Predisposing, Enabling, and Need Characteristics in Predicting Hospital, Physician, and Dentist Use

	Relative Importance		
Component	Hospital	Physician	Dentist
Predisposing			
Demographic	Medium	Medium	Medium
Social Structure	Low	Medium	High
Health Beliefs	Low	Low	Low
Enabling			
Family Resources	Medium	Medium	High
Community Resources	Low	Low	Low
Need			
Perceived	High	High	High
Evaluated	High	High	High

Source: Andersen, R.M., and Newman, J.F. (1973). Societal and Individual determinants of medical care utilization in the United States. *Milbank Memorial Fund quarterly* 51:95–124. Reprinted by permission.

Building on these revisions, Aday and Andersen (1974, 1975) introduced somewhat greater changes by expanding the model so that it could serve as a framework for the study of access to medical care. They (1974) conceptualize this framework as:

> proceeding from health policy objectives through the characteristics of the health care system and of the populations at risk (inputs) to the outcomes or outputs: actual utilization of health care services and consumer satisfaction with these services. (pp. 211–212)

Figure 3.5 portrays the interrelationships among the five blocks of factors that comprise their framework.

In the figure, health policy refers principally to the various programs that have been introduced to enhance and obtain equity in access. The characteristics of the health delivery system are essentially the same as the health services system in the Andersen and Newman (1973) revision. The characteristics of the population at risk is equivalent to the Andersen and Newman revision as well, with the exception that the illness level component is once again called need, and to facilitate policy discussions the dimensions of the predisposing and enabling components are now classified as mutable and immutable. The use of health services is equivalent to that identified in the Andersen and Newman revision as well. It is the introduction of

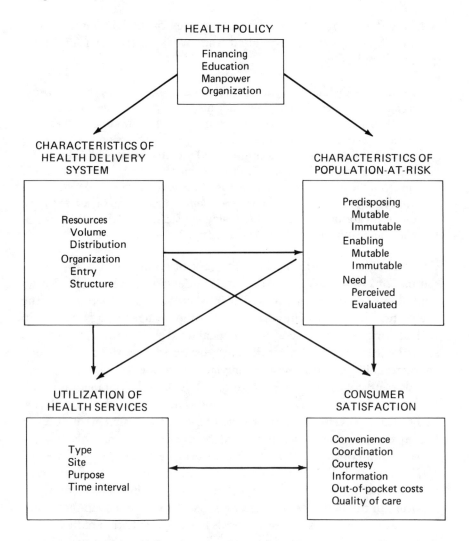

Figure 3.5 Framework for study of access to medical care.
Source: Aday, L. A., & Andersen, R. M. (1975). *Access to medical care.* Ann Arbor: Health Administration Press. Reprinted by permission.

consumer satisfaction (in addition to the formalization of health policy) that is new. It differs from the health-beliefs dimension of the predisposing component in that it represents the individual's satisfaction with the amount and quality of health care actually received. As such it adds something of a quality control (or assurance) dimension to the model.

Using data from a 1982 telephone survey of 4,800 families, Aday et al. (1984) applied the expanded framework to address four strategic health policy questions:

> 1) Have steady improvements in the access of traditionally disadvantaged groups such as minorities and the poor . . . continued into the 1980s? 2) Are there special access problems which traditional measures of access . . . fail to reveal? 3) Have the recession and high unemployment rates . . . accompanied by cutbacks in public health care programs and private health insurance coverage stymied or reversed the improving access trends of earlier periods. . . . 4) What are the implications for achieving or maintaining equity of access to medical care in the face of increasing constraints on the economy and the health care delivery system? (pp. 101–102)

Central to these questions is the concept of equity. When applied to the use of health services, Aday and Andersen (1981) argue that an equitable situation is one in which only medical need determines the use of health services (in addition to some vestiges of a relationship with age and sex, as proxies of biological need). In contrast, inequity is said to exist when health services are distributed on the basis of such characteristics as race, income, or place or residence.

Aday and colleagues (1984) found that 90% of the population have a regular source of care. This has not changed much since the early 1970s. Eighty-three percent of those surveyed reported spending 30 minutes or less in the physician's waiting room before being seen. This actually represents a considerable reduction in average waiting time since the 1970s. About 10% of the sample was without any form of public or private health insurance. That figure is also quite similar to those reported in the mid-1970s, suggesting that the poorer economic conditions of the late 1970s and early 1980s had not resulted in reducing this dimension of access to medical care. Thus, Aday and colleagues (1984) were left to conclude that the answers to the four health care policy questions presented earlier were favorable.

Others, however, would disagree. Mechanic (1985) suggests that access to health care for the poor, the elderly, and other disadvantaged groups has been eroding during the mid-1980s. He also considers their access to be particularly vulnerable to further declines in the face of the current budgetary crisis. Indeed, Berki et al. (1985) have shown that the economic hardships of the early 1980s disenfranchised many of the unemployed and underemployed from traditional private and public health insurance programs. Moreover, Wolinsky et al. (1987) have argued that the case for equity is not established simply because medical need is the best determinant of the use of health services, even in the absence of any other significant predictors (such as race, income, or health insurance). Noting that Aday et al. (1984) were able to explain less than 25% of the variance in the use of health services, Wolinsky et al. (1987) suggest that until more is known about why people use health services, it is premature to declare the health care delivery system to be equitable. Despite these concerns, the expanded behavioral model remains the dominant approach in the assessment of health and the use of health services.

Applications of Model to Elderly

Ward (1978, 1985) has argued that the behavioral model is particularly relevant for use in studying the use of health (and social) services of the elderly subpopulation. He notes two important reasons why. First, the model identifies mutable factors that facilitate the discussion and formation of public policy. Second, significant correlations exist between the sociodemographic factors and the use of health services among the elderly. Thus, Ward argues that gerontological health services research could significantly benefit from the adoption of the behavioral model.

Despite this enthusiasm, Ward (1978) also identifies two important shortcomings in applying the behavioral model to the special case of the elderly. The first of these involves the failure to consider how organizational factors associated with the bureaucratic nature of service delivery settings can serve as a barrier to use. In particular, Ward (1978) notes that:

> Older people, who seem to develop increased cautiousness and fatalism, may have difficulty penetrating bureaucratic service organizations, and have particular difficulty with fragmented systems which require active pursuit of services. . . . [O]rganizations represent a "culture" which may be supportive, neutral, or antagonistic to the culture of target groups. The culture may constitute a barrier to service utilization because of misfitting expectations, differential ordering of priorities, ego-assault in the professional-client encounter, or the prejudices of health professionals. (p. 67)

The second shortcoming is that social networks are not given much of a role in the behavioral model. Because research on the elderly has shown that these networks contribute significantly to the decision to use health services, Ward argues that the "lay referral" system needs to be included.

Similarly, McKinlay (1985) and Wolinsky et al. (1983) also raise some issues about the straightforward application of the behavioral model to the special case of the elderly. They express some concern that demographic models may not be as appropriate as psychosocial models for the aged population (see also Rakowski & Hickey, 1980). In a somewhat different vein, Wolinsky and Coe (1984) suggest (and present preliminary evidence to the effect) that the utility of the behavioral model's economic component may have become too limited since the advent of Medicaid and Medicare. That is, they posit that these federal entitlement programs may have leveled much of the discriminating ability of socioeconomic status.

Nonetheless, the behavioral model has become the dominant paradigm for studying the health and health behavior of the elderly. Indeed, during the 1980s several important studies have used the behavioral model (e.g., Branch et al., 1981; Evashwick, Rowe, Diehr, & Branch, 1984; Eve, 1982, 1984, 1988; Eve & Friedsam, 1980; Haug, 1981; Russell, 1981; Wan, Odell, & Lewis, 1982; Wolinsky, Arnold, & Nallapati, 1988; Wolinsky & Coe, 1984; Wolinsky et al., 1983). In general, these studies find that: (a) the need characteristics are the major determinants of the use of health services; (b) the amount of variance explained by the model is not large; and, (c) the regression coefficients obtained for the predisposing and enabling characteristics are modest, if not substantively unimportant. Moreover, the behavioral model has explained less of the variance in the elderly's use of health services than it has for the general population in the United States.

The principal explanation for the lower predictive utility of the behavioral model has been that the predisposing and enabling characteristics may no longer be important in the elderly's use of health services. Most health services (e.g., physician and hospital services) are now commonly covered by private or public health insurance programs. Thus, the salience of the predisposing and enabling characteristics has been eroded, although the cost-containment efforts begun in the late 1970s may be restoring the importance of these factors. Snider (1980a, 1980b), however, has suggested that the behavioral model may be more successful in predicting the use of ancillary services by adults. These services typically: (a) encompass more health maintenance or preventive health care than is the case with physicians and hospitals; (b) are more relevant to the needs of the elderly than formal acute-care services; and, (c) are less likely to be covered by insurance policies or included in outreach programs. Coulton and Frost (1982) provide some evidence to support Snider's interpretation.

Wolinsky and colleagues (see Wolinsky & Coe, 1984; Wolinsky et al., 1983) have taken a different approach. They argue that the limited predictive utility of the behavioral model among the elderly stems from measurement and modeling issues. On the measurement side, they note that most studies have not included comprehensive sets of indicators of the predisposing, enabling, and need characteristics. Particularly absent have been measures of the health care delivery system to which the elderly had access. In studies of the general population, Dutton (1978) and Kronenfeld (1978) have shown that the nature of the delivery system has marked effects on the use of health services.

Building on Mechanic's (1979) work, Wolinsky et al. (1983) also argue that restricted-activity and bed disability days represent illness behavior more than illness. As such, they should be considered measures of the use of health services, albeit in an informal sense. This argument is based on the fact that a person's taking of a restricted-activity or bed disability day usually involves both the provisional validation of the sick role by the individual's lay referral group (see Suchman, 1965) and the initiation of some form of self-treatment (such as the consumption of over-the-counter medications, especially among the elderly [see Denton, 1978]).

On the modeling side, Wolinsky and Coe (1984) have argued that the poor predictive utility of the behavioral model may also be a result of distortions introduced by the non-normally distributed indicators of the use of health services. Specifically, they note that the extreme positive skew observed in most utilization data significantly attenuates the assessment of the behavioral model in parametric analyses. As a corrective technique, Wolinsky and Coe suggest truncating the positive skew at the point where the curve becomes exceedingly flat (somewhere around the 95th percentile, or at about 13 visits to the physician, or 15 nights spent in the hospital, per person per year). This has the effect of reclassifying the most excessive users of health services as merely heavy users of health services.

Finally, although not specifically concerned with the use of health services by the elderly, two other alternative explanations have been offered for the poor predictive abilities of the behavioral model. Rundall (1981) focuses on the poor translation of the verbal (written) theory into mathematical estimations. He notes that although the model was originally (and continues to be) cast in interactive or conditional terms, it has always been estimated in an additive fashion. Thus, Rundall argues that it has never really had a fair test. Taking a somewhat different tack, Beland (1988) focuses on the way in which the use of health services is measured. He suggests that instead of counting the number of visits in a particular catchment period, it would be better to determine the interval between visits (i.e., consider each visit as a separate event) and then apply proportional hazards (or survival) models to the data. Although Beland (1988) presents some intriguing preliminary evidence, his approach requires knowing the date on which each health service was used. This information is seldom available in major health care surveys, such as the HISs.

REGRESSION-BASED COHORT ANALYTIC TECHNIQUES

An extended discussion of the principles, methods, and problems of traditional cohort analysis was contained in Chapter 1. It need not be repeated. Instead, the focus here is on the application of regression-based techniques to move beyond the general model reflected in Tables 1.1 to 1.4, and Equations 1.3 and 1.4. Specifically, two new approaches are presented. The first involves a method to obtain more precise estimates of the effects of age, period, and cohort. The second focuses on a method to assess whether the effects of the predisposing, enabling, and need characteristics are themselves affected by age, period, or cohort effects.

More Precise Estimates of Age, Period, and Cohort Effects

As shown in Chapter 1, the traditional approach to cohort analysis involves the construction and visual inspection of standard cohort tables (see Glenn, 1977). Regardless of how carefully one follows the guidelines for implementing those methods (see Glenn, 1976; Palmore, 1978), such analyses are rather limiting. The fundamental reason is that they essentially represent an examination of the unadjusted mean values of the variable of interest within each cell of the standard cohort table. That is, they (at least implicitly) assume that no factors other than age, period, and cohort affect the variable of interest. If such other factors exist, they can only be dealt with in traditional cohort analysis by standardization. This involves the introduction of a weighting algorithm that compensates only for the unequal distribution of those other factors across the cells of the table.

Moreover, it is difficult to standardize the distribution on more than a few variables simultaneously.

The tenuous nature of such assumptions can readily be demonstrated by recalling the example of the standard cohort table shown in Table 1.1. In it, the variable of interest was the percentage of respondents to public opinion polls who expressed a "great deal" of interest in politics. Surely, sex, race, political party affiliation, income, and religious preference would have had some effect here (see Pomper, 1976). Unless the data in Table 1.1 were simultaneously standardized to all of these factors, however, the results of the cohort analysis would be the logical equivalent of bivariate relationships between each of the explicitly identified effects (i.e., age, period, and cohort) and having a "great deal" of interest in politics.

Moreover, as sophisticated as the accounting formula presented by Mason and colleagues may be (see Feinberg & Mason, 1978; Mason & Fienberg, 1984; Mason, Mason, Winsborough, & Poole, 1973; Smith, Mason, & Fienberg, 1982), it also fails to go beyond the estimation of cell means unadjusted for anything but the other two of the three (i.e., age, period, and cohort) effects. The accounting formula, however, can be readily expanded to take such other factors into consideration. If O represents the set of other variables that are theoretically believed to influence whether one has a "great deal" of interest in politics, then the accounting formula can be rewritten as shown in Equation 3.1:

$$Y = k + \sum_{i=1}^{I-2} a_i A_i + \sum_{j=1}^{J-1} p_j P_j +$$

$$\sum_{k=1}^{K-1} c_k C_k + \sum_{l=1}^{L} o_l O_l + e \tag{3.1}$$

where Y is having a "great deal" of interest in politics, k is the intercept, A is the set of dummy variables representing the age categories and the a_i are their regression coefficients, P is the set of dummy variables representing the different periods and the p_j are their regression coefficients, C is the set of dummy variables representing the various birth cohorts and the c_k are their regression coefficients, O is the set of other variables of interest and the o_l are their regression coefficients, and e is the error or disturbance term. In Equation 3.1, the a_i, p_j, and c_k have become not just the effects of age, period, and cohort *net* among themselves, but *net* among themselves *and* of the set of other variables. Similarly, the effects of the o_i are *net* of each other *and* of the effects of age, period, and cohort. Unfortunately, this expansion adds to the complexities of estimating and interpreting the results of the accounting formula.

An alternative is to abandon the accounting formula altogether. In its place substitute the estimation of a multivariate regression equation within each column (i.e., period) of the standard cohort table. Table 3.3 contains an example of such a table that reflects the eight-cohort-by-four-survey design used in this study. (Note that because dental contact was not measured in the 1984 or 1985 HISs, only three columns are in this table.) The (dependent) variable of interest here is a dichotomy measuring whether or not the respondent had been to the dentist in the past 12 months. Age is measured by a set of dummy variables representing each of the nine cohorts through time. (Note that for convenience, any cohort that enters or leaves the standard table is designated as cohort 9.) Cohort 1 is the reference category, with its dummy variable omitted from the regression analysis. The other variables in the equation are standard indicators of the predisposing, enabling, and need characteristics of the individual. Shown in the table are the partial, unstandardized regression coefficients.

Within columns of Table 3.3 the interpretation of the cohort dummies is equivalent to the cross-sectional cohort assessment made within columns of traditional cohort tables. That is, comparisons of the regression coefficient for cohort 2 in 1972 to 1973 with that of any other cohort in 1972 to 1973 represents an age-strata comparison. Inasmuch as age-strata comparisons involve both the effects of cohort and age, the isolation of either of them necessarily must depend on the detection of the other. This inability to directly obtain a pristine cohort effect represents the most limiting aspect of this alternative approach.

The interpretation of the cohort dummies across columns (i.e., within rows) in Table 3.3 represents the change in the effect of belonging to a particular cohort as that cohort ages. This is a more pristine distillation of aging effects than that shown in the diagonal comparisons of standard cohort tables (such as Tables 1.1 to 1.4) for two reasons. First, the aging effects shown here are net effects, with the joint effects of the predisposing, enabling, and need characteristics having already been partitioned out. This has the added benefit of controlling for any compositional change effects associated with the predisposing, enabling, or need characteristics. Second, the multiple-

Table 3.3 Unstandardized Regression Coefficients (and Their Standard Errors) Obtained by Predicting Dental Contact During Past Year, for All Cohorts Combined, by Survey Year*

Independent variables	Survey years		
	1972-73	1976-77	1980-81
PREDISPOSING			
Demographic			
Sex	.040 (.005)	.042 (.005)	.035 (.005)
Widowhood	-.063 (.007)	-.072 (.008)	-.060 (.008)
Social Structure			
Education	.024 (.001)	.026 (.001)	.028 (.001)
Black		-.025 (.010)	
Hispanic			.065 (.017)
Labor force			
Living alone	.088 (.007)	.098 (.008)	.088 (.008)
ENABLING			
Family			
Income	.078 (.003)	.101 (.003)	.142 (.005)
Telephone	.058(.009)	.094 (.011)	.088 (.013)
Community			
Northeast	.040 (.006)	.027 (.007)	.031 (.007)
South	.029 (.006)	.031 (.006)	
West	.060 (.007)	.065 (.008)	.045 (.008)
Farm	-.025 (.010)		-.037 (.014)
Central city	.023 (.005)	.015 (.005)	
NEED			
Limited activity		-.015 (.006)	-.012 (.006)
Perceived health	.032 (.006)	.040 (.006)	.039 (.006)
COHORT STRUCTURE			
Cohort 2	-.022 (.007)		-.026 (.009)
Cohort 3	-.035 (.008)	-.048 (.009)	-.034 (.009)
Cohort 4	-.061 (.008)	-.062 (.009)	-.059 (.011)
Cohort 5	-.089 (.009)	-.094 (.011)	-.092 (.013)
Cohort 6	-.119 (.010)	-.113 (.013)	-.154 (.017)
Cohort 7	-.152 (.012)	-.161 (.017)	-.188 (.026)
Cohort 8	-.163 (.017)	-.149 (.027)	-.210 (.049)
Cohort 9	-.203 (.022)		.020 (.007)
Intercept		-.077 (.015)	-.103 (.017)
R^2	.139	.150	.153
N of Cases	41,093	36,230	35,588

*Coefficients not significantly different from 0 at the .05 probability level or beyond are omitted for clarity.

Source: Wolinsky, F.D., and Arnold, C.L. (1989). A birth cohort analysis of dental contact among elderly Americans. *American Journal of Public Health* 79:47–51. Reprinted by permission.

regression design is such that the associated period effects have been residualized to the intercept. Therefore, any differences observed by comparing, for example, the partial, unstandardized regression coefficient of cohort 2 in column 1 with that shown for it in column 2 reflect the effect of cohort 2's having aged 4 more years.

Similarly, this approach allows for a more pristine assessment of the period effects as well. They can be observed by comparing the intercept obtained from the equation estimated in column 1 with the intercept obtained from the equations estimated in columns 2 and 3. Because of the presence of the cohort dummies in the regression equations, these period comparisons are net of cohort effects, which confound period comparisons in standard cohort tables. Moreover, they are net of any compositional changes associated with the predisposing, enabling, and need characteristics because those are also represented in the regression equations.

This alternative approach to expanding the accounting formula has an important benefit in addition to its ability to provide direct estimates of the net effects of aging and period, and indirect estimates of the net impact of cohort. It allows the effects of the predisposing, enabling, and need characteristics to be compared across periods. This facilitates an evaluation of the stability of their effects over time. For example, compare the regression coefficient for income in column 1 with that for income in columns 2 and 3. They clearly indicate that income became more important as the decade of the 1970s gave way to the decade of the 1980s. This finding has important implications for assessing the equity of oral health care policy (see Wolinsky & Arnold, 1988b).

Assessment of Age, Period, and Cohort Effects on Structural Coefficients

As innovative as the alternative approach described earlier is, however, it cannot address the issue of whether the effects of the predisposing, enabling, and need characteristics are themselves subject to age, period, or cohort effects. Underlying this issue is the traditional and tacit assumption that the effects of these factors do not change (a) within cohorts as the cohorts themselves age, (b) across cohorts as older cohorts are replaced by younger cohorts, or (c) from historical period to historical period. These tacit assumptions seem tenuous.

For example, consider the case of income. Is it reasonable to assume that the importance of income in going to see a physician remains constant during the life course? Probably not, inasmuch as liquid assets decrease with age (see Atkins, 1985; Torrey, 1985). Should the effect of income be expected to remain the same from period to period? Not likely, given the remarkable changes in health care financing during the past two decades (see Anderson, 1985). Should the importance of income be expected to remain constant across different cohorts? Again, probably not, given the different economic experiential heritage between baby boomers and children of the Great Depression (see Elder, 1974, 1975).

These assumptions about the stability of (or change in) the effects of the predisposing, enabling, and need characteristics can be assessed using the following technique. First, a multiple regression equation is assembled that reflects the behavioral model of the use of health services described earlier. For reasons that will readily become apparent, age is *not* included in this equation. Second, this equation is then estimated separately within each cell of the standard cohort table (such as Table 3.1). The partial, unstandardized regression coefficients for each variable in the behavioral model subsequently become the input data (in lieu of the traditional means) for a new set of standard cohort tables. As in traditional cohort analysis, these tables are then inspected visually and statistically to identify any aging, period, or cohort changes in the regression coefficients. Table 3.4 contains an example of such a table in which the cell entries are the partial, unstandardized regression coefficients for the effect of the degree of limited activity owing to health conditions on the number of visits to physicians during the past 12 months reported by respondents in the HISs.

Making the diagonal comparisons that reveal the aging effects demonstrates the utility of this approach. (Note that similar row and column comparisons can be made to demonstrate the utility of this approach for examining period and cohort induced changes as well.) As the data in Table 3.4 indicate, the effect of the degree of limited activity on the rate of physician use declines as the cohorts age. That is, as the cohorts grow older, the same amount of limited activity results in fewer visits to the doctor than it did when they were younger. Moreover, this pattern is consistent for all but the very oldest of the cohorts.

A closer inspection of these data, however, reveals a pattern within a pattern. Within any cohort string (i.e., diagonal), the decline in the

Table 3.4 Partial, Unstandardized Regression Coefficients (and Standard Errors) Obtained for Limited Activity From Predicting Number of Physician Visits During Past Year (among Those With Visits), by Survey Year and Age-Group

Age-group	Survey year		
	1972-73	1976-77	1980-81
56-59	-.93 (.06)		
60-63	-.80 (.06)	-.91 (.06)	
64-67	-.76 (.06)	-.86 (.06)	-.74 (.06)
68-71	-.64 (.06)	-.76 (.06)	-.59 (.06)
72-75	-.68 (.07)	-.78 (.07)	-.66 (.07)
76-79	-.53 (.08)	-.57 (.08)	-.52 (.08)
80-83	-.42 (.10)	-.54 (.10)	-.45 (.10)
84-87	-.29 (.14)	-.31 (.14)	-.33 (.13)
88-91		-.61 (.24)	-.36 (.22)
92-95			-.57 (.45)

Source: Wolinsky, F.D., Aronold, C.L., and Nallapati, I.V. (1988). Explaining the declining rate of physician utilization among the oldest-old. *Medical Care* 26:544-553. Reprinted by permission.

rate of physician use as a response to limited activity owing to health reasons increases as the cohorts approach and pass through octogenarian status. This finding is quite important, inasmuch as it suggests that the previously reported declining rate of physician use among the oldest-old (see Soldo & Manton, 1985; Wolinsky et al., 1986) may result from their accelerated decreased response to health-related limitations in activity (see Wolinsky et al., 1988).

OPERATIONALIZATION OF MODEL

As indicated earlier, the behavioral model of the use of health services developed and subsequently modified by Andersen and colleagues (see Aday & Andersen, 1974, 1975; Aday et al., 1980, 1984; Andersen, 1968; Andersen & Newman, 1973) has been selected as the conceptual framework that guides the regression-based cohort analysis. Inasmuch as the model has been described earlier in considerable detail, the focus here is on the data available in the HISs with which to operationalize it. The predisposing, enabling, and need characteristics are considered first, followed by the measures of the use of health services.

Predisposing, Enabling, and Need Components

There are three dimensions to the predisposing component of the behavioral model: demographic factors, social structure, and beliefs. The only demographic factor specified by Andersen and Newman (1973; see also Figure 3.4) that is not available in the HISs is past illness. Thus, the demographic dimension is measured here by sex and marital status. Sex is a dummy variable scored 1 for women and 0 for men. Because this study focuses on the elderly, marital status is represented by a dummy variable for widowhood (see Hyman, 1983). It is scored 1 for widowed individuals and 0 for those who are not currently widowed.

Only two of the indicators of social structure shown in Figure 3.4, religion and residential mobility, are not available in the HISs. Thus, the social structure dimension is measured here by education, race and ethnicity, occupation, and family size. Education is expressed as the midpoints, in years, of 13 detailed categories ranging from none (0) to postgraduate studies (17). Race and ethnicity are tapped by introducing two dummy variables, one for being black, and the other for being Hispanic. Both are scored 1 if the individual is a member of that group, and 0 if he or she is not. The dummy variable for whites has been omitted from the analysis and serves as the reference category. Occupation is represented in the model as a dummy variable for labor-force participation. It is scored 1 if the individual meets the Census Bureau's criteria for being gainfully employed outside of the home, and 0 if he or she does not. Because this study focuses on the elderly, family size is represented by a dummy variable for living alone (see Cafferata, 1987; Homan, Haddock, Winner, Coe, & Wolinsky, 1986). It is scored 1 if the individual lives alone, and 0 if he or she lives with others.

Unfortunately, no measures of health beliefs are available for use in the HISs. Although this is less than desirable, previous studies have failed to identify significant effects of general health beliefs on the use of health services (see Andersen, 1968; Berkanovic, Telesky, & Reeder, 1981; Wolinsky et al., 1983). Thus, the omission of health beliefs from this study is not likely to have much impact on the analysis. Nonetheless, caution will be used to interpret the import of the predisposing characteristics on the use of health services owing to the absence of the beliefs dimension.

The enabling component of the behavioral model has two dimensions: family and community resources. Unfortunately, the only indicator of family resources shown in Table 3.4 that is available in the HISs is income. It is coded in tens of thousands of 1979 dollar equivalents, based on the midpoints of 13 categories that ranged from none to more than $25,000 in the 1972 to 1981 HISs, and from none to more than $50,000 in the 1984 and 1985 HISs. Also included as a measure of family resources is a dummy variable for the presence of a telephone in the household. The reason for this is that in the HISs, telephone consultations with physicians are counted as physician visits. The telephone dummy variable is scored 1 if a telephone is present, and 0 if it is not.

Having no measures of health insurance or access to a regular source of care represents the greatest measurement error problem facing this study. The problem is somewhat diminished by the fact that when health insurance, access to a regular source of care, and income are all included in the same analysis, income has the largest net effect (see Andersen, 1968). Moreover, the problem is somewhat further diminished by the fact that most of the sample is eligible for Medicare. This problem, however, is not eliminated. Therefore, caution will be exercised in interpreting the effects of the family resources dimension of the enabling characteristics on the use of health services.

Among the indicators of the community resources dimension of the enabling characteristics, the HISs only contain data on the region of the country in which the respondent lives, and the rural-urban character of his or her place of residence. Region of residence is measured by a set of three dummy variables for the Northeast, Southern, and Western divisions of the Census Bureau. They are scored 1 if the individual lives there, and 0 if he or she does not. The dummy variable for the Midwestern division has been omitted from the analysis and serves as the reference category. Place of residence is measured by a set of two dummy variables for living on a farm, or in the central city of a Standard Metropolitan Statistical Area (SMSA).

Either place of residence has traditionally been assumed to have the most disadvantaged access to medical care. These measures are scored 1 if the individual lives there, and 0 if he or she does not. The dummy variable for residence in small towns or suburbs of SMSAs has been omitted from the analysis and serves as the reference category. Although the absence of indicators of the supply of health personnel and facilities, and of the price of health services is unfortunate, prior studies have not found them to have significant effects on the use of health services (see Andersen, 1968). Thus, their absence is unlikely to affect the outcome of the analysis.

Two dimensions are also shown in Figure 3.4 among the need (i.e., illness-level) characteristics: perceived and evaluated. Inasmuch as the HISs do not contain any usable measures of symptoms or diagnoses, this study relies on the two standard indicators of perceived health: disability and general health status. Following recent suggestions (see Wolinsky & Arnold, 1988), limited activity owing to health reasons is represented by a dichotomy. It is scored 1 if the individual has any such limitations, and 0 if he or she does not. Similarly, perceived health status is also represented by a dichotomy. It is scored 1 if the individual assesses his or her health as excellent or good, and 0 if he or she responds that it is poor or fair. Although the absence of measures of symptoms and diagnoses is unfortunate, the available measures of limited activity and perceived health status have been shown to have the greatest impact on the use of health services. Thus, the analysis is not likely to be adversely affected.

For convenience, Table 3.5 summarizes the coding algorithms and contains the means and standard deviations for all of the predisposing, enabling, and need characteristics for all of the years of the HISs combined (i.e., 1972, 1973, 1976, 1977, 1980, 1981, 1984, and 1985). The distributions shown in the table are consistent with those reported from other national and regional surveys (see Aday et al., 1980, 1984; Andersen, 1968). Therefore, they need not here be described further.

Use of Health Services

As shown in Figure 3.3, Andersen and Newman (1973) suggest that three factors be considered when measuring the use of health services: type, purpose, and unit of analysis. Although the HISs facilitate the consideration of type and unit of analysis, they do not permit a disaggregation of the reason why the services were used (i.e., preventive vs. restorative care). This represents a limitation common to

Table 3.5 Coding Algorithms, Means, and Standard Deviations of Predisposing, Enabling, and Need Characteristics

Indicator	Coding algorithm	Mean	Standard deviation
Predisposing Characteristics			
Sex	1 = Female 0 = Male	.56	.50
Marital status	1 = Widowed 0 = Not widowed	.25	.43
Education	Actual number of years	10.12	3.71
Black	1 = Yes 0 = No	.06	.24
Hispanic	1 = Yes 0 = No	.02	.13
Labor force participation	1 = Yes 0 = No	.32	.47
Lives alone	1 = Yes 0 = No	.22	.42
Enabling Characteristics			
Income	Tens of thousands of 1979 dollars	11.97	7.96
Telephone in the home	1 = Yes 0 = No	.95	.23
Northeast region residence	1 = Yes 0 = No	.25	.43
Southern region residence	1 = Yes 0 = No	.32	.47
Western region residence	1 = Yes 0 = No	.17	.38
Central city SMSA residence	1 = Yes 0 = No	.30	.46
Farm residence	1 = Yes 0 = No	.04	.19
Need Characteristics			
Perceived health	1 = Excellent or good 0 = Fair or poor	.70	.46
Limited activity owing to health	1 = Yes 0 = No	.37	.48

nearly all large-scale health studies (see Wolinsky & Arnold, 1988). Therefore, the analysis is not likely to be jeopardized by the inability to separate out the purpose of the visit.

Based on the suggestions of Wolinsky et al. (1983), measures of both informal and formal use of health services have been selected. The use of informal health services is represented by two dichotomous measures of the taking of restricted activity or bed disability days. They are defined as contact measures, and are scored 1 if the individual reports having taken any such days during the past 2 weeks, and 0 if he or she did not.

The use of formal health services is represented by several measures of the use of dentists, physicians, and hospitals. Dental use is measured by a dichotomous contact variable scored 1 if the individual had seen a dentist during the past 12 months, and 0 if he or she had not. Physician use is measured in two ways. The first is a dichotomous contact variable scored 1 if the individual had seen a physician during the past 12 months, and 0 if he or she had not. The second measure of physician use is an indicator of the volume of physician visits reported by the respondent. It is scored as the actual number of visits reported, with the upper end of the distribution truncated such that 13 or more visits are mathematically treated as 13 visits (see Wolinsky & Coe, 1984). In accordance with the most current modeling approaches, when this volume measure of physician utilization is used, those individuals with no reported visits are excluded from the analysis (see Wolinsky & Arnold, 1988).

Hospital use is measured in three ways. The first is a dichotomous contact variable scored 1 if the respondent had been hospitalized for at least one night during the past 12 months, and 0 if he or she had not. The second measure of hospital use is the actual number of hospital episodes that occurred during the last 12 months. When this measure is used, those individuals who were not hospitalized in the past 12 months are excluded from the analysis (see Wolinsky & Arnold, 1988). The third measure of hospital use is an indicator of the volume of nights spent in the hospital during the past 12 months. It is scored as the actual number of nights reported, with the upper end of the distribution truncated such that 15 or more nights are mathematically treated as 15 nights (see Wolinsky & Coe, 1984). Again, when this volume measure of hospitalization is used, those individuals with no reported nights are excluded from the analysis (see Wolinsky & Arnold, 1988).

For convenience, Table 3.6 summarizes the coding algorithms and contains the means and standard deviations for all of the informal and

Table 3.6 Coding Algorithms, Means, and Standard Deviations of Measures of Health Services Use

Indicator	Coding algorithm	Mean	Standard deviation
Informal health services			
The taking of restricted activity days in the past two weeks	1 = Yes 0 = No	.15	.36
The taking of bed disability days in the past two weeks	1 = Yes 0 = No	.07	.25
Dentists' services			
Having seen a dentist in the past year	1 = Yes 0 = No	.48	.50
Physicians' services			
Having seen a physician in the past year	1 = Yes 0 = No	.78	.42
Number of visits to the physician in the past year (among those with visits)	Actual number of visits	4.91	4.00
Hospitals' services			
Having been hospitalized during the past year	1 = Yes 0 = No	.16	.37
Number of hospital episodes in the past year (among those with episodes)	Actual number of episodes	1.39	.87
Number of nights spent in the hospital in the past year (among those with episodes)	Actual number of nights	8.78	4.97

formal measures of the use of health services for all of the years of the HISs combined (i.e., 1972, 1973, 1976, 1977, 1980, 1981, 1984, and 1985). The distributions shown in the table are consistent with those reported from other national and regional surveys (see Havlik et al., 1987). Therefore, they need not here be described further.

SUMMARY

This chapter has presented the overall design of the study. It began with a justification, both theoretical and methodological, for the eight-cohort-by-four-survey design to be implemented in data taken from the HISs. Then the behavioral model of the use of health services was discussed, including its original specification, subsequent modification, and relevance to the special case of the elderly. Two newly developed regression-based cohort techniques were then introduced. One provides estimates of the aging, period, and cohort effects net of the effects of the predisposing, enabling, and need characteristics contained in the behavioral model. The other facilitates the assessment of whether these characteristics are themselves affected by age, period, and cohort effects. Chapter 3 concluded with an overview of how the behavioral model would be operationalized using the data taken from the HISs.

REFERENCES

Aday, L. A., & Andersen, R. M. (1974). A framework for the study of access to medical care. *Health Services Research, 9,* 208–220.

Aday, L. A., & Andersen, R. M. (1975). *Access to medical care.* Ann Arbor: Health Administration Press.

Aday, L. A., & Andersen, R. M. (1981). Equity of access to medical care: A conceptual and empirical overview. *Medical Care, 19* (December Suppl.), 4–27.

Aday, L. A., Andersen, R. M., & Fleming, G. V. (1980). *Health care in the U.S.: Equitable for whom?* Beverly Hills: Sage Publications.

Aday, L. A., Fleming, G. V., & Andersen, R. M. (1984). *Access to medical care in the U.S.: Who has it, who doesn't.* Chicago: Pluribus Press.

Andersen, R. M. (1968). *A behavioral model of families' use of health services.* Chicago: Center for Health Administration Studies.

Andersen, R. M., & Newman, J. (1973). Societal and individual determinants of medical care utilization in the United States. *Milbank Memorial Fund Quarterly, 51,* 95–124.

Andersen, R. M., Smedby, B., & Anderson, O. W. (1970). *Medical care use in Sweden and the United States: A comparative analysis of systems and behavior.* Chicago: Center for Health Administration Studies.

Anderson, O. W. (1963). The utilization of health services. In H. Freeman, S. Levine,

& L. Reeder (Eds.), *Handbook of medical sociology* (pp. 366–406). Englewood Cliffs, NJ: Prentice-Hall.

Anderson, O. W. (1985). *Health services in the United States: A growth enterprise since 1875.* Ann Arbor: Health Administration Press.

Anderson, O. W., & Sheatsley, P. J. (1967). *Comprehensive medical insurance: A study of costs, use, and attitudes under two plans.* New York: Health Information Foundation.

Atkins, G. L. (1985). The economic status of the oldest old. *Milbank Memorial Fund Quarterly, 63,* 395–419.

Beland, F. (1988). Utilization of health services as events: An exploratory study. *Health Services Research, 23,* 295–310.

Bengston, V. L., Cutler, N. E., Mangen, D. G., & Marshall, V. (1985). Generations, cohorts, and relations between age groups. In R. Binstock & E. Shanas (Eds.), *Handbook of aging and the social sciences* (2nd ed.) (pp. 304–338). New York: Van Nostrand Reinhold.

Berkanovic, E., Telesky, C., & Reeder, S. (1981). Structural and psychological factors in the decision to seek medical care for symptoms. *Medical Care, 19,* 693–709.

Berki, S. E., Wyszewianski, L., Lichtenstein, R., Gimotty, P., Bowlyow, J., Papke, E., Smith, T., Crane, J., & Bromberg, J. (1985). Health insurance coverage of the unemployed. *Medical Care, 23,* 847–854.

Binstock, R. H. (1985). The oldest old: A fresh perspective or compassionate ageism revisited. *Milbank Memorial Fund Quarterly, 63,* 420–451.

Branch, L., Jette, A., Evashwick, C., Polansky, M., Rowe, J., & Diehr, P. (1981). Toward understanding elder's health service utilization. *Journal of Community Health, 7,* 80–92.

Brody, E. M. (1985). Patient care as normative family stress. *The Gerontologist, 25,* 19–29.

Butler, R. N. (1975). *Why survive: Being old in America.* New York: Harper & Row.

Cafferata, G. L. (1987). Marital status, living arrangements, and the use of health services by elderly persons. *Journal of Gerontology, 42,* 613–618.

California Medical Association. (1960). *Relative value studies, 1960.* San Francisco: California Medical Association.

Callahan, D. (1987). *Setting limits: Medical goals in an aging society.* New York: Simon & Schuster.

Coulton, C. C., & Frost, A. K. (1982). Use of social and health services by the elderly. *Journal of Health and Social Behavior, 23,* 330–339.

Denton, J. (1978). *Medical sociology.* Boston: Houghton Mifflin.

Department of Health and Human Services. (1975). *The National Health Interview Survey procedure, 1957–1974* (DHHS Publication No. 75-1311). Washington, DC: Government Printing Office.

Department of Health and Human Services. (1985). *The National Health Interview Survey design, 1973–84* (DHHS Publication No. 85-1320). Washington, DC: Government Printing Office.

Durkheim, E. (1933). *Suicide.* New York: Free Press.

Durkheim, E. (1951). *The division of labor in society.* New York: Free Press.

Dutton, D. (1978). Explaining the low use of health services by the poor: Cost, attitudes, or delivery systems? *American Sociological Review, 43,* 348–367.

Elder, G. H. (1974). *Children of the Great Depression.* Chicago: University of Chicago Press.

Elder, G. H. (1975). Age differentiation and the life course. *Annual Review of Sociology, 1,* 165–190.

Evashwick, C., Rowe, J., Diehr, P., & Branch, L. (1984). Factors explaining the use of health care services by the elderly. *Health Services Research, 19,* 357–382.

Eve, S. B. (1982). Use of health maintenance organizations by older adults. *Research on Aging, 4,* 179–203.

Eve, S. B. (1984). Age strata differences in utilization of health care services among adults in the United States. *Sociological Focus, 17,* 105–120.

Eve, S. B. (1988). A longitudinal study of use of health care services among older women. *Journal of Gerontology, 43,* M31–M39.

Eve, S. B., & Friedsam, H. J. (1980). Multivariate analysis of health care services utilization among older Texans. *Journal of Health and Human Resources Administration, 3,* 169–191.

Feldstein, P. J. (1964). Demand for medical care. In *The cost of medical care.* Chicago: American Medical Association.

Feinberg, S. E., & Mason, W. M. (1978). Identification and estimation of age-period-cohort models in the analysis of discrete archival data. *Sociological Methodology, 1980,* 1–67.

Glenn, N. D. (1976). Cohort analysts' futile quest: Statistical attempts to separate age, period, and cohort effects. *American Sociological Review, 41,* 900–904.

Glenn, N. D. (1977). *Cohort analysis.* Beverly Hills: Sage Publications.

Hagestad, G. O., & Neugarten, B. L. (1985). Age and the life course. In R. H. Binstock & E. Shanas (Eds.), *Handbook of aging and the social sciences* (2nd ed.) (pp. 35–61). New York: Van Nostrand Reinhold.

Haug, M. (1981). Age and medical care utilization patterns. *Journal of Gerontology, 36,* 103–111.

Havlik, R. J., Liu, B. M., Kovar, M. G., Suzman, R., Feldman, J. J., Harris, T., & Van Nostrand, J. (1987). *Health statistics on older persons, 1986* (DHHS Publication No. 87-1409). Washington, DC: Government Printing Office.

Homan, S. M., Haddock, C. C., Winner, C. A., Coe, R. M., & Wolinsky, F. D. (1986). Widowhood, sex, labor force participation, and the use of physician services by elderly adults. *Journal of Gerontology, 41,* 793–796.

Hsiao, W. (1988, June). *The development of a relative medical value scale: A preliminary report.* Paper presented at the annual meeting of the Association for Health Services Research, San Francisco.

Hyman, H. (1983). *Of time and widowhood.* Durham, NC: Duke University Press.

Ibrahim, M. A. (1983). An epidemiologic perspective on health services research. In T. Choi & J. Greenberg (Eds.), *Social science approaches to health services research* (pp. 105–124). Ann Arbor: Health Administration Press.

Kronenfeld, J. (1978). Provider variables and the utilization of ambulatory care services. *Health Services Research, 19,* 68–76.

Maddox, G. W. (1979). Sociology of later life. *Annual Review of Sociology, 5,* 113–135.

Mason, W. H., & Fienberg, S. E (Eds.). (1984). *Cohort analysis in social research: Beyond the identification problem.* New York: Springer-Verlag.

Mason, K. O., Mason, W. H., Winsborough, H. H., & Poole, W. K. (1973). Some methodological issues in cohort analysis of archival data. *American Sociological Review, 38,* 242–258.

McKinlay, J. B. (1972). Some approaches and problems in the study of the use of services: An overview. *Journal of Health and Social Behavior, 13,* 115–152.

McKinlay, J. B. (1985, September). *Health care utilization by the elderly: Special considerations, methodological developments, and theoretical issues.* Paper presented at the invitational workshop on Aging and Formal Health Care. Jointly sponsored by the National Institute on Aging and the National Center for Health Services Research, Bethesda, MD.

Mechanic, D. (1978). *Medical sociology: A comprehensive text* (2nd ed.). New York: Free Press.

Mechanic, D. (1979). Correlates of physician utilization: Why do major multivariate studies of physician utilization find trivial psychosocial and organizational effects? *Journal of Health and Social Behavior, 20,* 387–396.

Mechanic, D. (1985). Cost containment and the quality of medical care: Rationing strategies in an era of constrained resources. *Milbank Memorial Fund Quarterly, 63,* 453–475.

Moore, W. E. (1969). Social structure and behavior. In E. B. Shelton & W. E. Moore (Eds.), *Indicators of social change* (pp. 27–46). New York: Russell Sage Foundation.

Mosely, R. R., & Wolinsky, F. D. (1986). The use of proxies in health surveys: Substantive and policy implications. *Medical Care, 24,* 496–510.

Newman, J. F. (1971). *The utilization of dental services.* Ph.D. dissertation, Emory University, Atlanta.

Palmore, E. (1978). When can age, period, and cohort be separated? *Social Forces, 57,* 285–295.

Parsons, T. (1951). *The social system.* New York: Free Press.

Parsons, T. (1958). Definitions of health and illness in light of American values and social structure. In E. G. Jaco (Ed.), *Patients, physicians, and illness* (pp. 120–144). New York: Free Press.

Parsons, T. (1975). The sick role and the role of the physician reconsidered. *Milbank Memorial Fund Quarterly, 53,* 257–278.

Paul, J. R. (1966). *Clinical epidemiology.* Chicago: University of Chicago Press.

Pomper, F. (1976). *The voters' choice.* New York: Dodd, Mead.

Rakowski, W., & Hickey, T. (1980). Late life health behavior: Integrating health beliefs and temporal perspectives. *Research on Aging, 2,* 3–20.

Rosenstock, I. (1966). What research in motivation suggests for public health. *American Journal of Public Health, 50,* 295–302.

Rosenthal, G. (1964). *The demand for general hospital facilities.* Chicago: American Hospital Association.

Rosow, I. (1985). Status and role change through the life cycle. In R. H. Binstock & E. Shanas (Eds.), *Handbook of aging and the social sciences* (2nd ed.) (pp. 62–93). New York: Van Nostrand Reinhold.

Rundall, T. (1981). A suggestion for improving the behavioral model of physician utilization. *Journal of Health and Social Behavior, 22,* 103–104.

Russell, L. (1981). An aging population and the use of medical care. *Medical Care, 19,* 633–643.

Smith, H. L., Mason, W. H., & Fienberg, S. E. (1982). More chimeras of the age-period-cohort accounting framework. *American Sociological Review, 47,* 787–793.

Snider, E. (1980a). Awareness and use of health services by the elderly: A Canadian study. *Medical Care, 18,* 1177–1182.

Snider, E. (1980b). Factors influencing health services knowledge among the elderly. *Journal of Health and Social Behavior, 21,* 371–377.

Soldo, B. J., & Manton, K. G. (1985). Changes in the health status and service needs of the oldest old: Current patterns and future trends. *Milbank Memorial Fund Quarterly, 63,* 286–323.

Stoeckle, J. M., Zola, I. K., & Davidson, B. (1963). On going to see the doctor, the contribution of the patient in the decision to seek medical aid. *Journal of Chronic Diseases, 16,* 975–989.

Suchman, E. (1965). Social patterns of illness and medical care. *Journal of Health and Human Behavior, 6,* 2–16.

Theodore, C. N. (1966). *The demand for health care services.* Unpublished M.A. thesis, Department of Economics, University of Illinois at Urbana, Illinois.

Torrey, B. B. (1985). Sharing increasing costs on declining income: The visible dilemma of the invisible aged. *Milbank Memorial Fund Quarterly, 63,* 377–394.

Wan, T. T. H. (1988). Antecedents of health services utilization in the older population. In M. Ory & K. Bond (Eds.), *Aging and the use of formal care* (pp. 52–78). New York: Routledge.

Wan, T. T. H., Odell, B., & Lewis, D. (1982). *Promoting the well-being of the elderly.* New York: Haworth Press.

Ward, R. (1978). Services for older people: An integrated framework for research. *Journal of Health and Social Behavior, 18,* 61–70.

Ward, R. (1985). *The aging experience* (2nd ed.). New York: Harper & Row.

Wirick, G. (1966). A multiple equation model of demand. *Health Services Research, 1,* 301–346.

Wolinsky, F. D. (1988). *The sociology of health: Principles, practitioners, and issues* (2nd ed.). Belmont, CA: Wadsworth.

Wolinsky, F. D., & Arnold, C. L. (1988). A different perspective on health and health services utilization. *Annual Review of Gerontology and Geriatrics, 8,* 71–101.

Wolinsky, F. D., & Arnold, C. L. (1989). A birth cohort analysis of dental contact among elderly Americans. *American Journal of Public Health, 79,* 47–51.

Wolinsky, F. D., Arnold, C. L., & Nallapati, I. V. (1988). Explaining the declining rate of physician utilization among the oldest-old. *Medical Care, 26,* 544–553.

Wolinsky, F. D., & Coe, R. M. (1984). Physician and hospital utilization among elderly adults: An analysis of the health interview survey. *Journal of Gerontology, 39,* 334–341.

Wolinsky, F. D., Coe, R. M., Miller, D. K., Prendergast, J. M., Creel, M. J., & Chavez, M. N. (1983). Health services utilization among the noninstitutionalized elderly. *Journal of Health and Social Behavior, 24,* 325–337.

Wolinsky, F. D., Coe, R. M., & Mosely, R. R. (1987). The use of health services by elderly Americans: Implications from a regression-based cohort analysis. In R. Ward & S. Tobin (Eds.), *Health in aging: Sociological issues and policy directions* (pp. 106–132). New York: Springer.

Wolinsky, F. D., Mosely, R. R., & Coe, R. M. (1986). A cohort analysis of the use of health services by elderly Americans. *Journal of Health and Social Behavior, 27,* 209–219.

Zola, I. K. (1964). Problems for research—Some effects of assumptions underlying sociomedical investigations. In G. Gordon (Ed.), *Proceedings, conference on medical sociology and disease control* (pp. 202–247). Chicago: Center for Health Administration Studies.

Chapter 4

Traditional Cohort Analysis

The purpose of this chapter is to present the results of the traditional cohort analysis of all of the measures of health and health behavior. It is divided into three major sections. The first focuses on the health status measures. This includes the respondent's perceived health status, and whether or not there are limitations to normal activities resulting from health problems. In the second section the focus is on the measures of the use of informal health services. This involves the number of days during the past 2 weeks in which the respondent's health problems have resulted in the taking of restricted activity or bed disability days. In the third section measures of the use of formal health services are considered. This includes contact and volume measures of dentist, physician, and hospital use.

In all of the traditional analyses reported in this chapter, the visual inspection of the standard cohort tables for aging, period, and cohort effects is governed by the following rule, in addition to those already discussed in Chapter 1. Differences between the means in any two (or more) comparative cells are considered to be significant only if the mean from the target cell falls outside of the 95% confidence interval(s) of the mean(s) of the comparison cell(s). That is, to be significantly different, the target mean must lie more than 2 standard errors away from the comparison mean. This ensures that any differences to

be discussed are meaningful differences and not those occurring simply because of sampling variance, which increases as sample sizes
decrease. Accordingly, any consistently observed significant patterns
should represent real aging, period, or cohort phenomena.

HEALTH STATUS

As indicated in Chapter 3, two measures of health status are available
in HISs. One is the traditional measure of perceived or subjective
health assessment. Before the 1982 HIS, respondents were asked to
say whether their health was excellent, good, fair, or poor. Since then,
respondents have been asked to say whether their health was excellent, very good, good, fair, or poor. In this study those responses were
then recoded into a dichotomous measure coded 1 when the response
was excellent, very good, or good, and 0 when it was fair or poor.

The second measure of health status is the traditional measure of
limitations in one's usual and major (i.e., work, school, etc.) activity
owing to health reasons. This information is derived by the inter-
viewer from a series of questions asked of the respondent. The
derived indicator has four categories: no limitations in activity, limitations affecting outdoor activities only, limitations affecting the
amount and kind of activities that can be performed, and limitations
so severe that usual and major activities cannot be performed at all.
Beginning with the 1982 HIS, a slight modification was introduced in
the construction of this index. Since then, the referent for respondents older than age 70 has been changed from one's usual and major
activities, to activities pertaining to personal daily living, regardless of
one's usual and major activities. In this study, the four response
categories have been recoded into a dichotomous measure coded 1
when any limitations in activity owing to health reasons were reported, and 0 when the respondent's activity was not limited in any
way. Because of the instrumentation change introduced in 1982,
special consideration will be given to the detection of an artificial
change associated with that period.

Perceived Health Status

Table 4.1 contains the results of the traditional cohort analyses of the
perceived health status measure. As indicated in Chapter 1, the effects
of aging can be seen by examining intracohort differences, or by
reading diagonally down and to the right. Such visual inspection of

Table 4.1 Proportion (and Standard Error) of Respondents Rating Their Health as Either Excellent or Good, by Survey Year and Age-Group

Age-group	Survey year			
	1972-73	1976-77	1980-81	1984-85
56-59	.735 (.004)	.743 (.005)	.751 (.005)	.766 (.005)
60-63	.705 (.005)	.696 (.005)	.712 (.005)	.726 (.005)
64-67	.692 (.005)	.695 (.006)	.699 (.006)	.702 (.006)
68-71	.693 (.006)	.692 (.006)	.680 (.006)	.684 (.006)
72-75	.678 (.007)	.682 (.007)	.681 (.007)	.669 (.007)
76-79	.652 (.008)	.681 (.008)	.676 (.009)	.655 (.008)
80-83	.655 (.010)	.681 (.010)	.686 (.010)	.631 (.011)
84-87	.665 (.015)	.650 (.015)	.688 (.014)	.625 (.014)
88-91	.714 (.022)	.702 (.022)	.682 (.023)	.661 (.021)
92-95	.734 (.039)	.702 (.042)	.754 (.039)	.620 (.041)
96-99	.667 (.083)	.742 (.080)	.783 (.061)	.500 (.082)

Table 4.1 indicates a generally uninterrupted decline in perceived health status before each cohort's reaching their early to mid-80s. That is, as these cohorts age, their members believe that their health gets worse. Once the cohorts' members reach their 90s, however, their perceived health status appears to stabilize. Further declines, if they occur, are at least not perceived by them. Both of these patterns hold regardless of whether one compares each cohort at successive 4-year intervals, or at the beginning and end of the study period.

These patterns are and are not consistent with an earlier and preliminary report based on this study (see Wolinsky, Mosely, & Coe, 1986). The similarity involves the first three columns and eight rows of Table 4.1, which were all that had been available earlier. These data show the generally uninterrupted decline in perceived health status as the six youngest cohorts aged. It is only after the fourth column and last two rows of Table 4.1 are considered that the dissimilarity emerges. By expanding on the information in Table 4.1, the stabilization of perceived health status among those cohorts who have reached their 90s becomes apparent. This underscores the importance of the expanded design used herein.

Although diagonal comparisons reflect aging effects, such visual inspections of standard cohort tables are confounded by the fact that they also reflect period effects. Accordingly, before the aging effects described earlier can be taken with great confidence, an assessment must also be made of the period effects. This is facilitated by reading across the rows. Such comparisons yield a somewhat more complex pattern consisting of three elements. The first element involves a slow increase in the perceived health status of the preretirement (i.e., 55- to 63-year-old) age-groups. This is entirely consistent with the well-documented improvements in health and life expectancy levels that have been experienced during the past two decades, as indicated in Chapter 2. The second element of this pattern involves the relatively stable perceptions of health status among younger-elderly (i.e., those 64 to 79 years old). This suggests that there has been virtually no period effect on the young-old during the 1970s and 1980s. The final element of this pattern involves those age-groups aged 80 or older. Among these groups of older-elderly a slow downward drift in perceived health status is palpable only if comparisons are made between the beginning and end points of the study period.

When taken together, these three elements of the pattern of period effects likely reflect the internalization of changing societal assessments of the elderly. Given the increasing social awareness of issues related to aging, the increase in perceived health status among the preretirement age-groups may reflect the recognition that people do not necessarily retire because of health reasons. Similarly, the stabilization in perceived health status among the young-old age-groups may reflect the recognition that people of this age generally are not faced with major limitations because of health problems. The gradual period decline associated with those age-groups aged 80 or more may reflect the increase in tabloid thinking that identifies the oldest-old as the reason for the increase in Medicare expenses and, thus, for much of the growing federal deficit (see Binstock, 1985). Regardless of the interpretation of these period effects, it is important to note that they do not in any way obfuscate the aging effects observed in the diagonal comparisons. Therefore, those aging effects stand.

Just as diagonal comparisons reflect both aging and period effects, row comparisons reflect both period and cohort effects. Thus, it is necessary to consider cohort effects before confidence can be expressed in the preceding identification of period effects. This is facilitated by making column comparisons of the data shown in Table 4.1. Such comparisons yield a two-part pattern. On the one hand, a general decline in perceived health status occurs as one progresses from the youngest cohorts to those cohorts in their early 70s by the early 1970s. Conversely, a general stabilization in perceived health status occurs as one progresses to the oldest cohorts. This means that those cohorts born during the 20th century perceive their health to be better than those in the 19th century, and that among those born in the 20th century, the most recently born perceive their health to be better than those less recently born.

Although this two-part pattern of cohort effects has no impact on the period effects described earlier, it is subject to aging effects, inasmuch as column comparisons involve both (i.e., cohort and aging effects). When the aging effects described earlier are juxtaposed, the resulting pattern is one of aging and not cohort effects. As a result, the traditional cohort analysis of perceived health status shown in Table 4.1 can be said to consist of both the aging and period effects discussed earlier, in the absence of any cohort effects.

Limited Activity

Table 4.2 contains the results of the traditional cohort analyses of the limited activity measure. The effects of aging can be seen by examining the intracohort differences, or by reading diagonally down and to the right. A remarkably strong pattern of aging effects can be seen here, although two factors blur that pattern somewhat. The general pattern, however, is that as these elderly cohorts age, more of their members incur some degree of activity limitations owing to health reasons. This occurs regardless of whether one compares each cohort at successive 4-year intervals, or at the beginning and end of the study period. It reflects the progressive physiological decline associated with age among the elderly that has been extensively documented (see Chapter 2) and is entirely consistent with the previous preliminary report from this study (see Wolinsky et al., 1986).

Table 4.2 Proportion (and Standard Error) of Respondents Having any Activity Limitations Owing to Health Reasons, by Survey Year and Age-Group

Age-group	Survey year			
	1972-73	1976-77	1980-81	1984-85
56-59	.256 (.004)	.269 (.005)	.274 (.005)	.278 (.005)
60-63	.309 (.005)	.328 (.005)	.338 (.005)	.333 (.006)
64-67	.350 (.005)	.365 (.006)	.385 (.006)	.395 (.006)
68-71	.385 (.006)	.409 (.006)	.420 (.007)	.354 (.006)
72-75	.443 (.007)	.449 (.007)	.453 (.008)	.349 (.007)
76-79	.502 (.008)	.486 (.009)	.494 (.009)	.378 (.008)
80-83	.540 (.011)	.531 (.011)	.557 (.011)	.447 (.011)
84-87	.595 (.015)	.621 (.015)	.606 (.015)	.527 (.015)
88-91	.665 (.023)	.651 (.023)	.659 (.023)	.636 (.021)
92-95	.711 (.040)	.661 (.043)	.683 (.042)	.676 (.039)
96-99	.788 (.072)	.839 (.067)	.761 (.064)	.842 (.060)

The principal factor in the blurring of this pattern involves an instrumentation artifact effect for all cohorts that reach or surpass their early 70s by the mid-1980s (i.e., the fourth column of the table). That represents the first HISs under examination in this study for which the activity referent was changed, as described earlier, from usual and major activities (such as work) to personal activities of daily living. Because the latter can generally be performed more readily in the presence of health problems than the former, a period effect in the form of a downward shift for all cohorts as they enter the fourth column of the table (when all of the cohorts are aged 70 years or more) is to be expected. The second issue that blurs the general pattern of aging effects is the fact that the period effect occurring in the fourth column of the table does not hold for all cohorts. Indeed, among the three oldest cohorts no artificial decline occurs. This most likely results from the rather small sample sizes (and thus larger standard errors) available for these oldest cohorts.

Confidence in this interpretation of aging effects depends on the verification of the period effects associated with the mid-1980s change in instrumentation. This is facilitated by reading across the rows to focus explicitly on the period effects. Such a visual inspection of the data in Table 4.2 reveals supporting evidence. A three-part pattern associated with the fourth column is readily detectable. It involves an increase in the degree of limited activity over time for those age-groups under 70 years old, a decline in limited activity over time for those age-groups in their early 70s to late 80s, and virtually no change over time for those age-groups in their 90s. It seems clear that the decline associated with those age-groups in their 70s and 80s reflects the change in instrumentation reflected in the mid-1980s HISs, and that the lack of change for those age-groups in their 90s reflects the rather small sample sizes available. What is not immediately intuitive is what the increase in limited activity for those age-groups under age 70 reflects. Because most of this is associated with changes between columns 1 and 2, it suggests that the explanation has something to do with preretirement policies and perceptions in the early 1970s.

Inasmuch as row comparisons reflect both period and cohort effects, column comparisons must be made before confidence can be expressed in the preceding interpretations. The data in Table 4.2 convincingly exhibit what appears to be a clear pattern of cohort effects. Older cohorts report higher mean levels of limited activity than younger cohorts, with two exceptions. The first exception involves the bottom two or three comparisons in each column, wherein no meaningful differences are detectable. This, again, is likely due to the small size of the available samples for these oldest age-groups. The second exception involves the third and fourth comparisons in the fourth column. One of these indicates no difference, whereas the other indicates a decrease in limited activity levels. Because these are two isolated occurrences, they likely reflect either statistical artifacts or particular historical factors associated with the mid-1980s.

In any event, the apparent dominant pattern based on column comparisons is that older cohorts report higher levels of limited activity. This provides further evidence that the period effects resulting from the change in instrumentation are in fact period effects rather than cohort effects. Moreover, because column comparisons reflect both cohort and aging effects, and in the absence of any demonstration of confounding period effects, the aging effects reflected in the diagonal comparisons suggest that the cohort effects described earlier are artifacts of the aging process. That is, when the three sets of comparisons are taken together, the evidence overwhelmingly supports the aging and period effects described earlier, but not the cohort effects. The latter appear only because of the confounding net effect of the aging process.

USE OF INFORMAL HEALTH SERVICES

As indicated in Chapter 3, two measures of the use of informal health services are available in the HISs. These are the number of days during the 2 weeks preceding the interview that the respondent's usual activities were restricted because of health reasons, and the number of days during that same period that the respondent was confined to bed owing to health reasons. In this study, those responses were then recoded into dichotomous measures coded 1 if one or more such days occurred, and 0 if no such days occurred.

Before proceeding to the traditional cohort analyses of these measures, further discussion seems warranted regarding their designation as indicators of the use of informal health services. The justification for this designation originates from Mechanic's (1979) seminal article on why large-scale multivariate analyses based on Andersen's (1968) behavior model fail to find anything but trivial effects for psychological and organizational factors on the use of health services. In that article, Mechanic focused directly on what has traditionally been considered to be appropriate indicators of illness behavior. After reviewing two decades of research, he found that the proponents of the behavioral model consider items such as restricted activity and bed disability days to be measures of the need characteristics. In contrast, Mechanic considers such items to be measures of illness behavior more appropriately. His argument is that these items represent the individual's behavioral response to perceived symptoms and the illnesses that underlie them.

Building on this approach, Wolinsky et al. (1983) noted that an important, additional reason existed for viewing items such as restricted activity and bed disability days as measures of illness behavior among the elderly. They observed that besides being responses to perceived symptoms, these items may well represent the first stage in the consumption of health services, albeit at an informal or nonprofessional level. That is, a person's taking of a restricted activity or bed disability day usually involves both the provisional validation of the sick role by the individual's lay referral group (see Suchman, 1965a, 1965b) and the initiation of some form of self-treatment, such as the consumption of over-the-counter medications (see Denton, 1978; Wolinsky, 1988). This is especially likely with the elderly as shown by the increased number of pharmaceutical remedies reportedly found in their homes (see Cape, Coe, & Rossman, 1983). It seems reasonable, therefore, to consider restricted activity and bed disability days as indicators of the use of informal health services.

Restricted Activity Days

Table 4.3 contains the results of the traditional cohort analyses of the restricted activity days measure. An examination of the aging effects, facilitated by reading diagonally down and to the right, fails to indicate any consistent patterns associated with the aging process. Rather, what can be observed is a consistent increase in the taking of restricted activity days as each cohort (except the oldest) ages 4 years between the early and mid-1970s, and a consistent decrease as each cohort (except the three oldest) ages 4 years between the early and mid-1980s. When intracohort comparisons are made between the beginning and end of the study periods, no pattern of change can be detected at all.

Because the observable effects occur only in the second and third columns, they likely reflect period effects rather than aging effects. It is most plausible that they respresent the impact of different economic conditions in the nation as a whole. More prosperous conditions during the mid-1970s likely resulted in both a greater sense of job and financial security that may have facilitated the taking of restricted activity days. In contrast, the more difficult economic times of the mid-1980s may have constrained the taking of restricted activity days, except among the oldest-elderly, who are least likely to be gainfully employed. In any event, the changes revealed from the diagonal comparisons are not indicative of aging effects.

Table 4.3 Proportion (and Standard Error) of Respondents Having Any Restricted Activity Days in Past 2 Weeks, by Survey Year and Age-Group

Age-group	Survey year			
	1972-73	1976-77	1980-81	1984-85
56-59	.136 (.003)	.148 (.004)	.158 (.004)	.126 (.004)
60-63	.138 (.004)	.154 (.004)	.163 (.004)	.118 (.004)
64-67	.141 (.004)	.148 (.004)	.161 (.004)	.127 (.004)
68-71	.146 (.005)	.164 (.005)	.173 (.005)	.122 (.004)
72-75	.152 (.005)	.170 (.006)	.173 (.006)	.137 (.005)
76-79	.163 (.006)	.173 (.007)	.184 (.007)	.145 (.006)
80-83	.168 (.008)	.180 (.008)	.187 (.009)	.160 (.008)
84-87	.194 (.012)	.195 (.012)	.177 (.011)	.152 (.011)
88-91	.174 (.018)	.200 (.020)	.181 (.019)	.156 (.016)
92-95	.242 (.038)	.165 (.034)	.183 (.035)	.155 (.030)
96-99	.242 (.076)	.194 (.072)	.174 (.057)	.132 (.056)

Considerable support for the period-effects interpretation is found by reading across the rows in Table 4.3. The beginning and end of study comparisons indicate that with the exception of the 80 to 83, 88 to 91, and 96 to 99 year-old age-groups, significant declines occur in the taking of restricted activity days. Comparisons of the same age-group at successive periods indicates that the overall decline results from the changes that occur between the early and mid-1980s. With the exception of the three oldest cohorts (whose members are least likely to be gainfully employed, and for whom the sample sizes are rather limited), significant declines occur at this point for all age-groups. When coupled with the diagonal comparisons, these row comparisons identify a significant period effect associated with the mid-1980s. In the absence of changes in instrumentation, this probably reflects the declining economic conditions described earlier.

Because row comparisons reflect both period and cohort effects, it is important to make the column comparisons to have confidence in the preceding interpretation. Doing so reveals that little is occurring with Table 4.3 that might be considered indicative of cohort effects. Indeed, of the 40 column comparisons that can be made, only 9 indicate a significant difference between successive age-groups. Even though these all indicate an increase in the taking of restricted activity days, they do not form or suggest any consistent pattern. That is, the differences do not consistently involve the same cohorts. Accordingly, the only meaningful effect that can be identified in Table 4.3 is a period effect associated with the increasing economic difficulties of the mid-1980s.

Bed Disability Days

Table 4.4 contains the results of the traditional cohort analyses of the bed disability days measure. An examination of the aging effects, facilitated by reading diagonally down and to the right, reveals an interesting but selective pattern. The pattern involves only cohorts 3 to 6, all of whose members fell into the young-old category (64 to 79 years of age) at the beginning of the study, and who were in the old-old category (76 to 91 years of age) at its conclusion. For these four cohorts, a significant increase occurs in the number of bed disability days as they age. Although this is not routinely evidenced from one period to the next for each of these cohorts, it is uniformly demonstrated as they age during the course of the study. This indicates that this aging effect is a relatively slow acting one. In contrast, no evidence of any aging effects, whether slow acting or not, is found for the preretirement, old-old, or oldest-old cohorts.

What might possibly account for such an aging effect restricted to those making the transition from young-old to old-old age status? Two factors seem plausible. The first involves a biological explanation and focuses on the increasing risk for health problems that results in the need for taking bed disability days. Confidence in such an explanation is somewhat shaken, however, by the fact that the literature indicates that such risk continues to progress into the 80s and beyond

Table 4.4 Proportion (and Standard Error) of Respondents Having Any Bed Disability Days in Past 2 Weeks, by Survey Year and Age-Group

Age-group	Survey year			
	1972-73	1976-77	1980-81	1984-85
56-59	.064 (.002)	.066 (.003)	.068 (.003)	.067 (.003)
60-63	.063 (.003)	.067 (.003)	.068 (.003)	.063 (.003)
64-67	.061 (.003)	.065 (.003)	.062 (.003)	.065 (.003)
68-71	.061 (.003)	.066 (.003)	.070 (.003)	.063 (.003)
72-75	.065 (.004)	.073 (.004)	.068 (.004)	.071 (.004)
76-79	.074 (.004)	.077 (.005)	.072 (.005)	.076 (.005)
80-83	.079 (.006)	.082 (.006)	.082 (.006)	.090 (.006)
84-87	.108 (.010)	.098 (.009)	.090 (.009)	.097 (.009)
88-91	.088 (.014)	.108 (.015)	.075 (.013)	.107 (.014)
92-95	.156 (.032)	.091 (.026)	.103 (.027)	.127 (.028)
96-99	.182 (.068)	.129 (.061)	.130 (.050)	.053 (.037)

(see Cape et al., 1983). Accordingly, it is not clear why this aging effect would be limited to the young-old.

The second explanation is more social and focuses on the changing role responsibilities associated with the life-course transitions that these young-old cohorts encounter. Being most likely to have retired from the labor force during this period, young-old men enjoy greater opportunities to take bed disability days without penalties or fear for their job security. With their men more likely to be retired and available at home to assist with household responsibilities, young-old women also enjoy greater opportunities to take bed disability days without risking significant disruption in domestic activites. The advantage of this explanation is that it is consistent with the limitation of this aging effect to the young-old. That is, it is plausible to assume that this social interpretation of the aging effect represents a transitional phase that stabilizes after adjustment to the new roles and obligations associated with being elderly.

Inasmuch as the diagonal comparisons reflect both aging and period effects, confidence in the preceding interpretation depends on the results of making the necessary row comparisons that might identify confounding period effects. Such row comparisons, however, indicate that nothing much is happening in Table 4.4. Indeed, of the 30 successive row comparisons that can be made, only 4 reveal significant differences. Moreover, only 2 of these occur in the same column (period), and they are in the opposite direction. Furthermore, comparisons of the beginning and end points of the study period uniformly fail to indicate any significant differences. Thus, considerable support is found for interpreting the diagonal differences as aging effects.

Similarly, confidence in the interpretation that no period effects exist depends on the column comparisons, inasmuch as cohort effects are also reflected in row comparisons. Like the row comparisons, the column comparisons indicate that nothing much is really happening in Table 4.4 in terms of cohort effects. Of the 40 possible successive column comparisons, only 5 indicate significant differences. Although all 5 show increases in the taking of bed disability days, no pattern can be identified. Indeed, no two of these increases involve the same cohort comparisons. Thus, the variation in the taking of bed disability days shown in the Table 4.4 is the result of the aging effect associated with the young-old.

USE OF FORMAL HEALTH SERVICES

As indicated in Chapter 3, there are six measures of the use of formal health services available in the HISs. These measures tap dentist, physician, and hospital use. The use of dentists' services is measured by a dichotomous contact measure. It is coded 1 if the respondent had been to see a dentist at some point during the 12 months preceding the interview, and 0 if he or she had not. Because of programmatic changes in the core data collection program of the HIS, the dental contact measure was not included in the 1984 and 1985 surveys.

Two measures of physician use are in this study. One is a contact measure that taps access to physicians. It is coded 1 if the respondent has seen any physician at least once during the 12 months preceding the interview, and 0 if he or she had not. The other measure reflects the volume of physician use. Consistent with current standards in the literature (see Chapter 3), the volume of physician use is calculated only among those with contact. This measure is coded as the actual number of visits, except that following Wolinsky and Coe (1984), it is truncated such that 13 or more visits are statistically treated (i.e., recoded) as 13 visits.

Similarly, hospital use is also measured in terms of contact and volume indicators. The contact measure is coded 1 if the respondent had been admitted for at least one night to a short-stay hospital during the 12 months preceding the interview, and 0 if he or she had not. Once again, the volume measures are calculated only among those who spent at least one night in the hospital. Here, however, there are two indicators of volume. One involves the actual number of hospital episodes (i.e., admissions) that occurred during the 12 months preceding the interview, and the other involves the actual number of nights spent in the hospital during the same period. As suggested by Wolinsky and Coe (1984), the volume of hospital use is truncated (i.e., recoded) such that 15 or more nights are statistically treated as 15 nights.

Dental Contact

Table 4.5 contains the results of the traditional cohort analyses of the dental contact measure. An examination of the aging effects, facilitated by reading diagonally down and to the right, does not reveal an entirely straightforward pattern. Indeed, those cohorts aged 60 to 75 years old at the onset of the study have relatively stable dental contact rates throughout. Only the youngest cohort shows a significant decline during the course of the study, and it is not consistent for both successive comparisons. The four oldest cohorts experience either a stable or modest increase between the early and mid-1970s, followed by a larger decline 4 years later. Because the change associated with the oldest cohorts all occurs between columns 2 and 3, it most likely reflects an interaction between aging and period effects such that in the early 1980s dental contact rates declined only for the oldest-old. Thus, the most consistent pattern among these diagonal comparisons is the absence of any aging effects.

Table 4.5 Proportion (and Standard Error) of Respondents Having Seen a Dentist During Past 12 Months, by Survey Year and Age-Group

Age group	Survey year		
	1972-73	1976-77	1980-81
56-59	.522 (.005)	.571 (.005)	.607 (.005)
60-63	.467 (.005)	.512 (.006)	.558 (.006)
64-67	.422 (.006)	.475 (.006)	.497 (.006)
68-71	.376 (.006)	.412 (.006)	.451 (.007)
72-75	.326 (.007)	.373 (.007)	.418 (.007)
76-79	.279 (.008)	.317 (.008)	.370 (.009)
80-83	.227 (.009)	.293 (.010)	.331 (.011)
84-87	.203 (.013)	.226 (.013)	.243 (.013)
88-91	.160 (.018)	.236 (.021)	.205 (.020)
92-95	.109 (.028)	.190 (.036)	.151 (.032)
96-99	.176 (.095)	.200 (.107)	.167 (.078)

A visual inspection of the row comparisons indicates what appears to be a consistent pattern of increasing dental contact rates. With three exceptions (involving the three oldest cohorts during the early 1980s), the successive comparisons reveal higher rates of dental contact over time. This pattern is uniformly reflected when the beginning and end points of the study are compared. Although this observation would be consistent with period effects reflecting the increasing relative supply of dentists, confidence in that interpretation must be considered tentative inasmuch as these row comparisons also contain cohort effects. Nonetheless, the fact that the dental contact rates for the three oldest cohorts decline in the early 1980s reaffirms the aging and period effect interaction described earlier.

Although further analyses are required to clarify the preceding interpretation of this interaction effect, it likely is related to the higher rate of inflation experienced during the late 1970s and early 1980s. It is plausible that such inflationary restraints would affect dental contact rates among the oldest-old the most (or solely). The reason is that the oldest-old have substantially less wealth and liquid assets than younger cohorts (see Atkins, 1985; Torrey, 1985; Wolinsky & Arnold, 1989). Therefore, they are more likely to be forced to make a choice between dental care and more essential goods and services.

The column comparisons reveal consistent age-group increases with only one exception (which indicates no change). When combined with the absence of any aging effects, this demonstrates that these age-group differences are due to cohort succession. Moreover, because such strong cohort effects have been isolated, the differences revealed from the row comparisons also likely result from cohort effects and not from aging effects. Indeed, the only major pattern occurring in Table 4.5 (other than the age and period interaction described earlier) is that of cohort succession. Older cohorts having lower dental contact rates are simply being replaced by younger cohorts having higher dental contact rates. The dental contact rates of the individual cohorts themselves are stable over time, being virtually unaffected by aging or period factors. These results, then, reflect the progressively increasing salience of both oral health and oral hygiene to successive birth cohorts.

Physician Use

Table 4.6 contains the results of the traditional cohort analyses of the physician contact measure. An examination of the diagonal comparisons reveals an interesting pattern of aging effects contained in three parts. The first part involves the overall increase in physician contact rates as the cohorts age. This is reflected in the rather consistent successive comparisons between the early to mid-1970s, and between the early to mid-1980s. It is also reflected by the fact that significant increases in physician contact are found during the entire study period for all but the two oldest cohorts. The second part of the pattern involves a period effect that apparently occurs between the second

Table 4.6 Proportion (and Standard Error) of Respondents Having Seen a Physician During Past 12 Months, by Survey Year and Age-Group

Age-group	Survey year			
	1972-73	1976-77	1980-81	1984-85
56-59	.712 (.005)	.755 (.005)	.740 (.005)	.737 (.005)
60-63	.717 (.005)	.754 (.005)	.755 (.005)	.761 (.005)
64-67	.727 (.005)	.763 (.005)	.750 (.005)	.791 (.005)
68-71	.739 (.006)	.792 (.005)	.785 (.005)	.810 (.005)
72-75	.759 (.006)	.801 (.006)	.801 (.006)	.827 (.006)
76-79	.765 (.007)	.792 (.007)	.810 (.007)	.829 (.007)
80-83	.761 (.009)	.787 (.009)	.806 (.009)	.851 (.008)
84-87	.777 (.013)	.795 (.012)	.794 (.012)	.843 (.011)
88-91	.726 (.022)	.757 (.021)	.802 (.019)	.837 (.016)
92-95	.664 (.042)	.711 (.041)	.730 (.040)	.796 (.034)
96-99	.606 (.086)	.774 (.076)	.674 (.070)	.789 (.067)

and third columns. That is, with one exception no significant changes occur in physician contact rates for any cohort between the mid-1970s and the early 1980s. The third part of the pattern is that for the two oldest cohorts (i.e., those who were 80 years old or older at the onset of the study), virtually no change in physician contact rates occurs.

This pattern is and is not consistent with an earlier preliminary report based on this study (see Wolinsky et al., 1986). The similarity involves the increase in physician contact associated with the aging of the six youngest cohorts. The dissimilarities involve the detection here of the apparent period effect occurring between columns 2 and 3, and the lack of any aging effect among those cohorts aged 80 years old or more at the onset of the study. Both of these could not be detected previously because that earlier report included neither the mid-1980s data nor the two oldest cohorts. By expanding on information in Table 4.6, however, the stabilization of physician contact among octogenarians becomes apparent, as does the continuation of the aging effect among the younger cohorts. The former is especially salient inasmuch as it suggests that the aging effect "tops-out" as the members of the cohorts become octogenarians. This is consistent with and lends further support to the inverse J-curve relationship with a pivotal point at about age 80 between age and the volume of physican visits that was identified earlier (see also Wolinsky, Arnold, & Nallapati, 1988; Wolinsky, Coe, & Mosely, 1987). Confidence in this pattern of aging effects, however, depends on whether the row comparisons indicate any period effects, which would also be reflected in the diagonal comparisons.

An examination of the row comparisons yields similarly mixed results. During the course of the entire study (i.e., from the early 1970s to the mid-1980s) an increase in physician contact rates occurs for all age-groups. For the four oldest age-groups, however, this increase is virtually undetectable when successive 4-year comparisons are made. In contrast, for those age-groups younger than their early 80s, the increase over time is detected in about two thirds of the successive comparisons. The weakest period changes occur between the mid-1970s and the early 1980s. Because these mixed results are so similar to those observed when making the diagonal comparisons, it is necessary to make the column comparisons to separate the effects of period from those of age.

The successive age-group comparisons within the columns indicate that, in general, little related to cohort phenomena is happening in Table 4.6. When significant differences do occur, they reflect increasing physician contact rates associated with age. This occurs until age-groups are compared that include individuals in their mid-80s. From that point on, decreasing physician contact rates are associated with increasing age. Thus, these column differences reflect age and not cohort effects.

Because of that, the row comparisons identified earlier reflect period and not cohort effects, which means that most (but not all) of the age-related differences revealed in the diagonal comparisons are indicative of period effects rather than aging effects. Nonetheless, when coupled with the age-related differences found in the diagonal comparisons, the observance of some aging effects in the column comparisons suggests that a modest level of aging effects do in fact exist.

In the end, then, it appears that the largest effects on physician contact rates are associated with historical change. Over time, physician contact rates have increased, although they have done so more for the younger cohorts than for the older cohorts. Smaller but nonetheless important aging effects were also found. They suggest that as cohorts age, their physician contact rates increase, until that time when the cohorts' members reach their eighth decade. At that point, physician contact rates appear to stabilize. These interrelated aging and period effects will be discussed further following the analysis of the volume of physician use.

Table 4.7 contains the results of the traditional cohort analyses of the volume of physician use among those who saw a physician at least once during the preceding 12 months. The diagonal comparisons indicate a two-part pattern of aging effects. First, among the four youngest cohorts no detectable aging effect exists. Indeed, only one successive comparison reveals a significant change, and it involves a decrease in the volume of physician use. None of these younger cohorts exhibits a significant change during the course of the entire study period.

The second part of the pattern involves a decline during the course of the study period among the three youngest of the four oldest cohorts. Because this change is concentrated in the comparisons involving columns 2 and 3, it might appear to be a period effect that only applies to the older-elderly. That interpretation is marginally enhanced by the fact that the only aging effect observed among the four youngest cohorts involved a decline in the volume of physician use for those aged 76 to 79 in the early 1980s. Thus, in the early 1980s a decline occurred in the volume of physician use for all cohorts who had aged into their mid-70s or beyond. If it could be substantiated, such an age-specific period effect would likely reflect increasing restrictions in the extent of ambulatory care coverage provided by Medicare that were introduced at that time. It is plausible that this would affect the old- and oldest-old more than the young-old because the latter have substantially greater economic wealth, and their assets are disproportionately more liquid (see Atkins, 1985; Torrey, 1985; Wolinsky & Arnold, 1989). Therefore, they would be more likely to be less dependent on and sensitive to restrictive

Table 4.7 Number of Physician Visits in Past 12 Months (and Standard Error) among Those With at Least One Visit, by Survey Year and Age-Group

Age-group	Survey year			
	1972-73	1976-77	1980-81	1984-85
56-59	4.876 (.049)	4.712 (.049)	4.437 (.049)	4.374 (.052)
60-63	5.025 (.052)	4.825 (.051)	4.605 (.050)	4.602 (.054)
64-67	5.225 (.056)	5.033 (.055)	4.854 (.055)	4.850 (.057)
68-71	5.432 (.062)	5.211 (.059)	4.998 (.059)	4.958 (.060)
72-75	5.643 (.070)	5.440 (.068)	5.149 (.067)	5.016 (.067)
76-79	5.796 (.083)	5.630 (.083)	5.212 (.081)	5.289 (.077)
80-83	5.754 (.106)	5.644 (.099)	5.322 (.100)	5.369 (.099)
84-87	5.891 (.151)	5.561 (.146)	5.187 (.131)	5.140 (.126)
88-91	5.388 (.229)	4.965 (.231)	5.006 (.210)	5.177 (.190)
92-95	5.400 (.453)	5.860 (.468)	4.446 (.405)	4.894 (.368)
96-99	7.400 (.953)	5.583 (.955)	4.677 (.716)	7.000 (.801)

changes in Medicare. Confidence in such an interpretation, however, depends on the corroboration of an age-specific period effect in the examination of the row comparisons.

An examination of the row comparisons yields an interesting two-part pattern of period effects. The first part involves the consistent overall decline in the volume of physician use among those age-groups under age 88. This decline holds for all eight of these age-groups during the course of the study period, and for all but two age-groups when

the successive comparisons are made involving the first three columns. No successive comparisons between the early and mid-1980s
yield significant differences.

The second part of the pattern of row comparisons is the virtual
absence of any significant differences among the age-groups including
the oldest-old. A comparison of the beginning and end points of the
study fails to detect any meaningful changes. The successive 4-year
comparisons indicate only two significant changes. One of these increases, whereas the other decreases. When taken together, these row
comparisons suggest a period effect such that a general decline in
physician use has occurred, but that it had slowed by the mid-1980s,
and that it did not alter the rate of physician use among the oldest-old.
This pattern fails to corroborate the age-specific period effect interpretation advanced earlier based on the diagonal comparisons.

It is only after the column comparisons are made, however, that the
overall patterns in Table 4.7 can be understood. Like the row comparisons, the column comparisons reveal a two-part pattern. On the one
hand, when the successive age-group comparisons are made for those
age-groups under age 80, consistent age-related increases in the volume of physician use are seen. Indeed, of the 20 such comparisons, 17
indicate significant increases. Conversely, when the successive age-
group comparisons are made for those age-groups older than age 80,
no consistent age-related changes occur in the volume of physician
use. Rather, of the 20 such comparisons here, only 6 indicate any
significant differences, with 4 reflecting declines and 2 reflecting
increases. Moreover, no cohort pattern can be detected among these
differences. This suggests that the column comparisons reflect aging
rather than cohort effects, but those aging effects, which reflect an
increase in the volume of physician visits, top-out if not actually begin
to reverse once the cohorts reach their 80s.

When taken together, then, the three sets of comparisons reveal the
following pattern of effects in Table 4.7. No cohort effects are occurring. In contrast, aging and period effects exist, and these are so
intertwined and offsetting as to form a rather complex pattern that is
not readily apparent from a casual visual inspection. On the one hand,
the period effects reflect a general decline over time in the volume of
physician use among those with contact. This much seems reasonably
straightforward. Conversely, the aging effects reflect an increase in
physician use as the cohorts age, until they reach their eighth decade.
At that point, their rate of physician use begins to decline. This effect
is masked in the diagonal comparisons by the offsetting period effects,
which are approximately equal in strength. As a result, the only

perceptible changes in the diagonal comparisons are those that occur after the cohorts reach age 80 or more, when their physician use rates actually begin to decline.

These results are not directly comparable with the previous and preliminary report from this study (see Wolinsky et al., 1986). Three reasons exist for this. One is that the earlier report did not restrict the analysis of the volume of physician use to those who had one or more visits. The other two are that the earlier report included neither the mid-1980s HISs (the last column in Table 4.7) nor the two oldest cohorts (the last two rows in Table 4.7). As a result, direct comparisons to that earlier report are not entirely appropriate. Nonetheless, the findings are similar.

At this point, an integration of the results of the traditional cohort analyses of the physician contact and volume of physician use measures is in order. Table 4.6 revealed an increase in physician contact rates over time (i.e., a period effect) that was stronger for the younger than for the older cohorts. This was coupled with a smaller aging effect such that as the cohorts aged, they were more likely to have at least one contact annually with a physician, with one exception. That exception was that the rate of physician contact appeared to stabilize as the cohorts' members became octogenarians. No plausible cohort effects were detected. Thus, it appeared that access to physicians' services, as indexed by contact rates, increased owing to a combination of age and period effects, but that this increase stabilized among the oldest-old.

Similarly, regarding the volume of physician use among those with contact, Table 4.7 revealed age and period but no cohort effects. The aging effect here was similar, resulting in an increase in physician use until the cohorts reached their eighth decade. At that point, the volume of their use began to decline. In contrast, however, the period effect revealed in Table 4.7 indicates a decline in the rate of physician use over time.

What can, then, plausibly explain these opposite period and consistent aging effects? The period effects are actually intuitively pleasing. At the same time that access to health care has been increasing during the 1970s and 1980s, cost-containment efforts and the increasing health of the population have reduced the average volume of physician use among those with access to physicians. The increase in access probably reflects both the expanding relative supply of physicians and the growing recognition that the early detection of chronic killer diseases (such as cancer) through annual checkups can greatly enhance survival rates. The decrease in the volume of physician use most likely results primarily from the greater fiscal constraints imposed by third-party insurers on follow-up visits.

Explaining the consistent aging effects on both the contact and volume rates of physician use is somewhat more difficult. This is because both increase with age, until the cohorts' members become octogenarians. At that point, physician contact rates stabilize, and the volume of physician use actually begins to decline. Therefore, there are two parts of the pattern to explain. The most likely explanation of both is that they correlate reasonably well with the aging effects shown in Tables 4.1 and 4.2 for the perceived health status and limited activity measures. Indeed, perceived health status consistently declined among all cohorts whose members were younger than 80 years old by the mid-1970s, but was relatively stable among those cohorts aged 80 years old or older. Similarly, although limited activity owing to health reasons increased as each cohort aged, that increase was much more gradual among the oldest cohorts. Thus, the increase in the contact and volume rates of physician use may well reflect increasing self-assessed need among the elderly up to age 80, at which point they see their needs as either stabilizing or actually decreasing, in a relative sense.

Such an interpretation contains both biological and social elements. The biological element explains the increase in physician contact and volume rates based on evaluated need, and is consistent with the literature documenting the physiological decline associated with aging (see Cape et al., 1983). The social element explains the stabilization in the physician contact rate and the decline in the volume of physician visits as octogenarians begin to redefine their health problems and limitations as merely accepted components of normal aging (see Ferraro, 1980). Accordingly, they begin to take less action (i.e., go to see a physician less often) in response to their health problems (see Wolinsky et al., 1988). This interpretation, however, must remain somewhat tentative until the more sophisticated regression-based cohort analytic techniques have been introduced in Chapter 5.

Hospital Use

Table 4.8 contains the results of the traditional cohort analyses of the hospital contact measure. An examination of the diagonal comparisons reveals a remarkably consistent pattern associated with the aging process. For all cohorts significant increases occur in hospital contact during the course of the study. Moreover, significant increases occur in hospital contact for all but four of the successive comparisons

Table 4.8 Proportion (and Standard Error) of Respondents Hospitalized during Past 12 Months, by Survey Year and Age-Group

Age-group	Survey year			
	1972-73	1976-77	1980-81	1984-85
56-59	.128 (.003)	.132 (.004)	.128 (.004)	.112 (.004)
60-63	.133 (.004)	.135 (.004)	.134 (.004)	.137 (.004)
64-67	.146 (.004)	.155 (.004)	.153 (.004)	.158 (.005)
68-71	.146 (.004)	.176 (.005)	.168 (.005)	.167 (.005)
72-75	.179 (.006)	.180 (.006)	.193 (.006)	.192 (.006)
76-79	.198 (.007)	.198 (.007)	.200 (.007)	.223 (.007)
80-83	.195 (.009)	.217 (.009)	.218 (.009)	.228 (.009)
84-87	.201 (.012)	.229 (.013)	.216 (.012)	.250 (.013)
88-91	.177 (.018)	.226 (.021)	.198 (.019)	.249 (.019)
92-95	.195 (.035)	.223 (.038)	.222 (.037)	.282 (.038)
96-99	.242 (.076)	.290 (.083)	.174 (.057)	.237 (.070)

within cohorts. The four successive comparisons that do not reflect a significant increase all occur among the oldest-old. Thus, these data indicate an aging effect that begins to slow down (but remains significant) among the oldest-old. This aging effect mirrors that observed for limitations in activity owing to health reasons (see Table 4.2). As such, it seems likely that the increase in hospital contact is due to the increase in limited activity.

The row comparisons associated with Table 4.8 reveal a gradual increase in the rate of hospital contact over time. Although this increase is shown for all but two of the 11 possible row comparisons during the course of the study, it is palpable for only 9 of the 33 possible successive comparisons. As such, this rather slow increase in the rate of hospital contact probably reflects the increasing relative supply of hospital beds, as well as the trend toward shorter average lengths of hospital stays that occurred during the 1970s and 1980s (see Department of Health and Human Services, 1985). Both of these social phenomena served to increase the opportunity for hospital episodes. The increase in hospital contact rates may also reflect the effect of the perverse incentive of the PPS that results in a focus on the generation of more hospital episodes, inasmuch as the basis of reimbursement has shifted from fee for service to episodes of care (see Wolinsky, 1988). In the absence of data from the late 1980s (after the effects of PPS would have been fully manifested), however, confidence in such an interpretation must remain tentative.

The column comparisons in Table 4.8 fail to indicate any significant pattern of cohort effects. Indeed, among those age-groups aged 84 years or more, only one successive comparison indicates any significant difference, and it is marginal. Among the younger age-groups the successive comparisons reveal significant differences 15 out of 24 times. All of these represent increases associated with age. Given the consistent and strong aging effects shown in the diagonal comparisons, however, it is most likely that these column comparisons reflect age and not cohort effects.

Table 4.9 contains the results of the traditional cohort analyses of the number of hospital episodes among those persons with at least one such episode during the past 12 months. A two-part pattern can be seen in the diagonal comparisons. The first is a gradual increase in the number of hospital episodes that is only palpable when the comparisons involve the beginning and end points of the study. Indeed, only 6 of the 24 successive comparisons yield significant differences. The second part of the pattern of aging effects is that they exist primarily only for the five youngest cohorts. Among the three oldest cohorts only one significant successive comparison exists during the course of the entire study. Thus, the aging effects appear to be relatively weak and confined to the younger cohorts.

Confidence in interpreting the preceding as aging effects, however, depends on the existence and nature of any period effects, inasmuch as both are involved in diagonal comparisons. Because most (4 out of 6) of the changes that can be observed in the diagonal successive comparisons occur between the early to mid-1970s, it is plausible to expect a historically limited period effect. The row comparisons do

Table 4.9 Number of Hospital Episodes (and Standard Error) During Past 12 Months among Those With at Least One Episode, by Survey Year and Age-Group

Age-group	Survey year			
	1972-73	1976-77	1980-81	1984-85
56-59	1.280 (.021)	1.288 (.024)	1.354 (.024)	1.413 (.034)
60-63	1.318 (.021)	1.323 (.021)	1.413 (.031)	1.427 (.027)
64-67	1.327 (.023)	1.367 (.026)	1.392 (.025)	1.475 (.034)
68-71	1.337 (.033)	1.382 (.025)	1.399 (.026)	1.422 (.030)
72-75	1.348 (.026)	1.348 (.026)	1.393 (.031)	1.441 (.031)
76-79	1.379 (.028)	1.361 (.029)	1.400 (.040)	1.448 (.035)
80-83	1.355 (.035)	1.384 (.043)	1.430 (.042)	1.447 (.040)
84-87	1.329 (.045)	1.442 (.054)	1.440 (.056)	1.433 (.047)
88-91	1.447 (.102)	1.330 (.070)	1.381 (.091)	1.445 (.077)
92-95	1.440 (.183)	1.519 (.235)	1.143 (.067)	1.450 (.107)
96-99	1.500 (.189)	1.222 (.147)	1.125 (.125)	1.444 (.242)

not support that suspicion, however. Only 5 of the 33 successive comparisons indicate significant differences, and only one of these occurs between the early to mid-1970s. Thus, it is unlikely that the aging effects identified earlier are the masked results of a historical artifact. At the same time, however, the row comparisons involving the 8 youngest age-groups during the entire course of the study do reveal significant increases in the number of hospital episodes among those with one or more such events. Because these gradual increases are so similar to those found in the diagonal comparisons, it is necessary to examine the column comparisons before a positive attribution of the effects can be made.

The column comparisons indicate that virtually nothing is occurring in terms of cohort effects in Table 4.9. Indeed, of the 40 successive comparisons that can be made, only one indicates a significant difference. When taken together, then, the column comparisons (which reflect both cohort and aging effects), the diagonal comparisons (which reflect both aging and period effects), and the row comparisons (which reflect both period and cohort effects) indicate that the variations shown in Table 4.9 result from period effects and not from aging effects. Over time a gradual increase in the number of hospital episodes has occurred among those with at least one, but virtually no such effect has occurred among the oldest age-groups. Such a period effect is consistent with the pattern of hospital contact described earlier. Between the early 1970s and the mid-1980s more individuals have been hospitalized, and they have been hospitalized more often. Both of these trends (i.e., period effects), however, have been rather slow. Although the trend for hospital contact was accompanied by an increase associated with the aging process, the trend for the number of hospital episodes was not.

Table 4.10 contains the results of the traditional cohort analyses of the number of nights spent in the hospital during the past 12 months among those spending at least one night there. An examination of the diagonal comparisons fails to reveal any consistent aging effects, even though significant declines are observed for cohorts 2 through 6 over the course of the entire study. Indeed, of the 24 successive comparisons that can be made, only 8 indicate significant differences. Although all of these reflect declines in the number of nights spent in the hospital, 6 of them occur in the last column of Table 4.10. Inasmuch as that column corresponds to the first 2-year period during which the PPS system (a major goal of which was to reduce average lengths of stay) was in place for Medicare patients, this probably represents a period rather than an aging effect.

An examination of the row comparisons supports such a period effects interpretation. For all but the two oldest age-groups, significant declines in the number of nights spent in the hospital are detected during the course of the entire study period. Gradual declines can be detected between the early 1970s and the early 1980s, although palpable consecutive declines during that period are rare. The successive cohort comparisons, however, indicate that most of the overall

Table 4.10 Number of Nights Spent in Hospital (and Standard Error) During Past 12 Months Among those With Hospital Episodes, by Survey Year and Age-Group

Age-group	Survey year			
	1972-73	1976-77	1980-81	1984-85
56-59	8.616 (.140)	8.311 (.143)	8.008 (.149)	7.617 (.171)
60-63	8.929 (.143)	8.888 (.150)	8.425 (.149)	8.048 (.161)
64-67	9.316 (.147)	8.975 (.147)	8.829 (.151)	8.313 (.159)
68-71	9.563 (.163)	9.574 (.154)	9.053 (.161)	8.433 (.160)
72-75	9.965 (.163)	9.848 (.170)	9.348 (.168)	8.543 (.174)
76-79	10.115 (.186)	9.701 (.188)	9.302 (.203)	8.402 (.185)
80-83	10.046 (.233)	9.555 (.224)	9.614 (.234)	8.639 (.239)
84-87	10.493 (.330)	10.012 (.318)	9.651 (.319)	8.547 (.293)
88-91	10.316 (.563)	9.979 (.518)	9.750 (.522)	8.711 (.431)
92-95	10.200 (.913)	8.259 (.863)	9.286 (.934)	9.725 (.756)
96-99	13.125 (1.076)	9.667 (1.667)	7.500 (1.899)	10.556 (1.930)

decline occurs between the early to mid-1980s (i.e., between columns 3 and 4). This adds confidence to the preceding interpretation that the variation in Table 4.10 likely reflects the effects of the PPS system. In particular, it suggests that physicians and hospitals were sensitive to the average lengths of stays targeted for each of the DRGs, and modified their practice patterns accordingly. Thus, it would appear that Medicare's shift to an episode-based capitation system was an effective cost-containment device, at least in terms of reducing the number of nights spent in the hospital.

The successive age-group comparisons within the columns of Table 4.10 indicate that not much is happening. Only 11 of the 40 possible such comparisons yield significant differences. Although all of these reflect age-related increases in the number of nights spent in the hospital, they do not form a consistent pattern with regard to age-group. Thus, apparently no cohort effects are occurring in Table 4.10. This finding lends further credence to the interpretation of the period effects associated with the implementation of the PPS system and its targeted lengths of stay for each DRG as being the only pattern of effects occurring in Table 4.10.

At this point an integration of the results of the traditional cohort analyses of the measures of hospital contact, episodes, and nights spent in the hospital is in order. No cohort effects were detected for any of these measures of hospital use. An aging effect was found only for the measure of hospital contact. As the members of these eight cohorts aged, the probability of their being hospitalized increased, although that increase began to slow down somewhat among the oldest-old. This pattern of aging effects is consistent with that observed for limited activity owing to health reasons, suggesting that the increase in hospital use is driven by an increase in need.

Significant period effects were found for all three measures of hospital use. Between the early 1970s and the mid-1980s more individuals have been hospitalized, and they have been hospitalized more often. This has been a gradual (or slow) trend that was difficult to detect consistently in successive comparisons. It was readily detectable, however, during the course of the entire study period. It probably reflects primarily the combined effects of the increasing relative supply of hospital beds and the shorter average lengths of stay that occurred during this period. Because these increases were so gradual (and not associated with any particular column), it is unlikely that they reflect at all the introduction of the PPS as part of Medicare.

In contrast, the period effect associated with the number of nights spent in the hospital seems tied to the introduction of the PPS as part of Medicare. Although a gradual decline can be detected between the early 1970s and the early 1980s, most of the period changes that can be detected here occur between the early to mid-1980s (i.e., between columns 3 and 4), when the targeted average lengths of stay for each of the DRGs was implemented. Thus, although the probability of hospitalization and the number of times one was likely to be hospitalized was gradually increasing, the number of nights spent in the hospital was gradually decreasing. That gradual decrease, however, turned into a palpably sharp decline with the implementation of the PPS in the mid-1980s.

SUMMARY

This chapter has presented the results of the traditional cohort analyses of all of the measures of health and health behavior. It began with the two measures of health status. These were the respondent's self-assessed health status and activity limitations owing to health reasons. Attention then shifted to the use of informal health services. The two measures examined here were the taking of restricted activity or bed disability days during the 2 weeks before the interview. In the final section six measures of the use of formal health services were considered. These included contact and volume measures of dentist, physician, and hospital use during the 12 months preceding the interview.

Three rather interesting patterns emerged. First, the only cohort effect that was detected involved dental use. Older cohorts having lower dental contact rates were simply being replaced by younger cohorts having progressively higher dental contact rates. No aging or period effects were involved in the process. Thus, those analyses were indicative of a classic case of pure cohort succession.

On the one hand, the fact that cohort effects were identified for only one of the 10 measures under study may indicate that there simply were no cohort effects other than those associated with dental contact. Conversely, it may indicate that although 4-year intervals are appropriate for detecting aging and period effects, they are not sufficiently sensitive for detecting cohort effects (except for dental contact). Only subsequent analyses using cohorts with wider age-bands can resolve that issue. Unfortunately, such analyses are not possible when using these HISs (unless a design with fewer than three time points [i.e., columns] is used). Thus, the issue cannot be further addressed in this study.

The second interesting pattern involved the aging effects. In general, health status declined as the cohorts aged, although that decline seemed to stabilize (for the perceived health status measure) or at least slow down (for the limited activity measure) among the oldest-old. For the most part, the only aging effect found among the use of informal health services involved the bed disability days measure. Here the effect was limited to those cohorts involved in the transition from young-old to old-old status. They experienced an increasing likelihood of taking bed disability days. Among the measures of the use of formal health services, aging effects were found for the contact measures of both physician and hospital use, as well as for the volume measure of physician use. The use of these formal health services increased as the cohorts aged, although this increase either decelerated, stabilized, or reversed itself as the cohorts aged into their eighth decade and beyond.

The third interesting pattern involved the period effects. They are not nearly so easy to summarize as were the cohort and aging effects. The self-assessed health of the preretirement age-groups got better over time. The perceived health of those age-groups aged 80 or older, however, slowly drifted downward during the course of the study. In contrast to the results for self-assessed health status, the degree of limited activity among the preretirement groups got worse over time. Aside from the instrumentation effect that occurred between the early to mid-1980s, no other period effects were detected for the activity limitations measure. Among the measures of the use of informal health services, the only detectable period effect involved the taking of restricted activity days. Over time, fewer such days were taken by most of the age-groups, with most of this change occurring between the early to mid-1980s.

As indicated earlier, no period effects were observed regarding dental contact. This was not the case, however, for physician use. Here, a two-part pattern emerged. Over time, contact with physicians increased for all age-groups, reflecting enhanced access to health care. At the same time, however, the volume of physician visits (among those with at least one visit) declined for all but the three oldest age-groups. Thus, it would appear that although access to physicians increased, restrictions were placed on the volume of services (most probably follow-up visits) that were allowed.

Like physician contact, hospital contact and the number of hospital episodes (among those having at least one such episode) increased for nearly all of the age-groups during the course of the study. These increases, however, were rather gradual and dispersed over time. They could seldom be detected by comparing successive 4-year periods. In contrast, the period effect on the number of nights spent in the hospital (among those with one or more episodes) resulted in a consistent decline. That decline was rather gradual until the mid-1980s when it sharpened considerably. That significant downturn parallels the implementation of the PPS on average lengths of stay among elderly patients.

REFERENCES

Andersen, R. M. (1968). A behavioral model of families' use of health services. Chicago: Center for Health Administration Studies.

Atkins, G. L. (1985). The economic stress of the oldest old. Milbank Memorial Fund Quarterly, 63, 395–419.

Binstock, R. H. (1985). The oldest old: A fresh perspective or compassionate ageism revisited. Milbank Memorial Fund Quarterly, 63, 420–451.

Cape, R. D. T., Coe, R. M., & Rossman, I. (Eds.). (1983). Fundamentals of geriatric medicine. New York: Raven Press.

Department of Health and Human Services. (1985). Charting the nation's health: Trends since 1960 (DHHS Publication No. 85-1251). Washington, DC: Government Printing Office.

Denton, J. (1978). Medical sociology. Boston: Houghton Mifflin.

Ferraro, K. L. (1980). Self-ratings of health among the old and old-old. Journal of Health and Social Behavior, 21, 377–382.

Mechanic, D. (1979). Correlates of physician utilization: Why do major multivariate studies of physician utilization find trivial psychosocial and organizational effects? Journal of Health and Social Behavior, 20, 387–396.

Suchman, E. (1965a). Social patterns of illness and medical care. Journal of Health and Human Behavior, 6, 2–16.

Suchman, E. (1965b). Stages of illness and medical care. Journal of Health and Human Behavior, 6, 114–128.

Torrey, B. B. (1985). Sharing increasing costs on declining income: The visible dilemma of the invisible aged. Milbank Memorial Fund Quarterly, 63, 377–394.

Wolinsky, F. D. (1988). The sociology of health: Principles, practitioners, and issues. Belmont, CA: Wadsworth.

Wolinsky, F. D., & Arnold, C. L. (1989). A birth cohort analysis of dental contact among elderly Americans. American Journal of Public Health, 79, 47–51.

Wolinsky, F. D., Arnold, C. L., & Nallapati, I. V. (1988). Explaining the declining rate of physician utilization among the oldest-old. Medical Care, 26, 544–553.

Wolinsky, F. D., & Coe, R. M. (1984). Physician and hospital utilization among elderly adults: An examination of the Health Interview Survey. Journal of Gerontology, 39, 334–341.

Wolinsky, F. D., Coe, R. M., Miller, D. K., Prendergast, J. M., Creel, M. J., & Chavez, M. N. (1983). Health services utilization among the noninstitutionalized elderly. Journal of Health and Social Behavior, 24, 325–336.

Wolinsky, F. D., Coe, R. M., & Mosely, R. R. (1987). The use of health services by elderly Americans: Implications from a regression-based cohort analysis. In R. Ward & S. Tobin (Eds.), Health in aging: Sociological issues and policy directions (pp. 106–132). New York: Springer Publishing Co..

Wolinsky, F. D., Mosely, R. R., & Coe, R. M. (1986). A cohort analysis of the use of health services by elderly Americans. Journal of Health and Social Behavior, 27, 209–219.

Chapter 5

Regression-Based Cohort Analysis

The purpose of this chapter is to present the results of the regression-based cohort analysis of all of the measures of health and health behavior. As such, the chapter is divided into two major sections. The first focuses on the more pristine assessment of the age, period, and cohort effects. These are obtained by estimating multivariate regression equations reflecting the behavioral model of the use of health services separately within each survey year. Using the comparative process described later, the resulting regression coefficients yield the *net* effects attributable to age, period, and cohort, as well as the *net* effects of the predisposing, enabling, and need characteristics.

In the second section the focus shifts to the assessment of aging, period, and cohort effects on the predisposing, enabling, and need characteristics themselves. This is accomplished by estimating the behavioral model separately for each cohort within each survey year. The resulting coefficients are then placed into standard cohort table formats. These are subsequently examined to reveal whether any particular effect, such as income, significantly varies across diagonal, row, or column comparisons.

In all of the regression-based cohort analyses reported here, the visual inspection of the tables for aging, period, and cohort effects is (again) governed by the following rule. Differences in the unstandardized regression coefficients in any two (or more) comparative cells are considered to be significant only if the coefficient from the target cell falls outside of the 95% confidence interval(s) of the coefficient(s) of the comparison cell(s). That is, to be significantly different, the target coefficient must lie more than 2 standard errors away from the comparison coefficient. This ensures that any differences discussed are meaningful, and do not occur simply because of sampling variance.

MORE PRISTINE ASSESSMENTS OF AGE, PERIOD, AND COHORT EFFECTS

Before proceeding to a discussion of the results shown subsequently in Tables 5.1 to 5.10, it would seem appropriate to briefly review how those results were obtained, and how they are to be interpreted. As indicated earlier, multivariate regression equations reflecting the behavioral model of the use of health services (see Chapter 3 for a detailed discussion of that model) were separately estimated within each survey year. Age was measured by a set of dummy variables representing each of the eight cohorts through time, with any cohort that enters or leaves the standard table arbitrarily designated as cohort 9. Cohort 1 was the reference category, with its dummy variable omitted from the regression analysis. The other variables included in the equation are the standard indicators of the predisposing, enabling, and need characteristics of the individual. Shown in the tables that follow are the partial, unstandardized regression coefficients and their standard errors.

Within columns of any of these tables the interpretation of the cohort dummies for cohorts 2 through 8 is equivalent to the cross-sectional cohort assessment made within columns of traditional cohort tables (see Chapter 4). For example, comparisons of the coefficient for cohort 2 in 1972 to 1973 with that of any other cohort in 1972 to 1973 represent age-strata comparisons. Note, however, that because cohort 9 is a residual cohort for those age-groups that either enter or leave the cohort table, it (and it alone) is not suitable for meaningful comparisons. Inasmuch as any age-strata comparisons involve both the effects of cohort and age, the isolation of either of them necessarily must depend on the detection of the other. The inability to obtain a pristine cohort effect directly represents the most limiting aspect of this regression-based approach.

The interpretation of the cohor dummies across columns (i.e., within rows) in these tables represents the change in the effect of belonging to a particular cohort as that cohort ages. This is a more pristine distillation of aging effects than that obtained from the traditional cohort analysis reported in Chapter 4 for two reasons. First, the aging effects shown here are *net* effects, with the joint effects of the predisposing, enabling, and need characteristics having been partitioned out. Second, the design is such that most of the associated period effect has been residualized to the intercept. Therefore, any differences observed by comparing, for example, the coefficient of cohort 2 in column 1 with that shown for it in column 2 more closely reflects the effect of cohort 2's having aged 4 more years.

Similarly, this approach allows for a more pristine assessment of the period effects as well. They can be observed by comparing the intercept obtained from the equation estimated in column 1 with that obtained in columns 2 through 4. Because of the presence of the cohort dummies in the regression equations, these period comparisons are net of cohort effects, which confounded period comparisons in the standard cohort tables presented in Chapter 4. Moreover, the period comparisons made subsequently are net of any compositional changes associated with the predisposing, enabling, and need characteristics because those are also represented in the regression equations.

Health Status

Table 5.1 contains the results of the regression-based cohort analysis of the perceived health status measure. The results show that the predisposing and enabling characteristics are able to explain 10.9% to 12.6% of the variance. Perceiving one's health to be excellent or good is positively related to being a woman, attaining education, participating in the labor force, living alone, having income, having a telephone, living in the Northeast (vs. living in the Midwest), and being a certain age. At the same time, perceived health status is negatively related to being black, living in the South (vs. living in the Midwest), or living on a farm (vs. living in a small city or suburb of an SMSA). For the most part, these relationships are replicated within each column of Table 5.1. They are also generally consistent with the extant literature on the elderly's self-assessed health status (see Ferraro, 1980; Fillenbaum, 1979).

Among the predisposing and enabling characteristics, however, significant and patterned changes in the magnitude of the effects for

Table 5.1 Unstandardized Regression Coefficients (and Their Standard Errors) Obtained by Predicting Perceived Health, for All Cohorts Combined, by Survey Year*

Independent variables	Survey years			
	1972-73	1976-77	1980-81	1984-85
PREDISPOSING				
Demographic				
Sex	.037 (.005)	.039 (.005)	.047 (.005)	.035 (.005)
Widowhood			-.015 (.007)	
Social structure				
Education	.018 (.001)	.018 (.001)	.020 (.001)	.018 (.001)
Black	-.045 (.008)	-.065 (.009)	-.072 (.009)	-.086 (.009)
Hispanic		.040 (.016)		
Labor force	.178 (.005)	.174 (.006)	.175 (.006)	.153 (.006)
Living alone	.082 (.007)	.087 (.007)	.081 (.007)	.091 (.007)
ENABLING				
Family				
Income	.056 (.002)	.073 (.003)	.101 (.004)	.148 (.006)
Telephone	.045 (.008)	.058 (.010)	.052 (.012)	.073 (.014)
Community				
Northeast		.014 (.006)	.019 (.006)	.019 (.007)
South	-.071 (.006)	-.062 (.006)	-.045 (.006)	-.031 (.006)
West			.024 (.007)	
Farm	-.053 (.010)	-.057 (.012)		
Central city				
COHORT STRUCTURE				
Cohort 2	.014 (.007)	.059 (.007)	.027 (.008)	
Cohort 3	.060 (.007)	.081 (.008)	.046 (.009)	
Cohort 4	.090 (.008)	.086 (.009)	.049 (.010)	
Cohort 5	.092 (.009)	.103 (.010)	.081 (.012)	
Cohort 6	.091 (.010)	.099 (.012)	.101 (.015)	
Cohort 7	.096 (.012)	.088 (.016)	.082 (.024)	
Cohort 8	.124 (.016)	.133 (.025)	.163 (.045)	
Cohort 9	.193 (.021)		-.040 (.006)	-.027 (.007)
Intercept	.292 (.012)	.254 (.013)	.245 (.015)	.217 (.017)
R^2	.109	.113	.126	.120
N of Cases	41,093	36,230	35,588	32,348

*Coefficients not significantly different from 0 at the .05 probability level or beyond are omitted for clarity.

five variables occur over time. These are being black, participating in the labor force, having income, living in the South (vs. living in the Midwest), and living on a farm (vs. living in a small city or suburb of an SMSA). The negative effect of being black increases over time. Indeed, the coefficient nearly doubles, indicating considerable growth in the racial gap in perceived health status between whites and blacks. This reflects the well-documented and increasing racial inequity in health status observed between blacks and whites (see Andersen, Mullner, & Cornelius, 1987; Manton, Patrick, & Johnson, 1987).

In contrast, the positive effect of working becomes less important over time. This change, however, is only palpable when the effect obtained in the mid-1980s is compared with that from any earlier period. When coupled with the fact that the coefficients for labor-force participation shown in columns 1 through 3 are nearly isomor-phic, the decline observed for column 4 probably represents more of an artifact than the beginning of a stable trend. Nonetheless, the drop-off is statistically significant.

The changes in the effect of income are substantial, consistent, and significant regardless of which column comparisons are made. Over time, the positive effect of income on perceived health status nearly triples. By the mid-1980s its effect is such that for every $10,000 increment in family income, older Americans are about 15% more likely to rate their health status as excellent or good versus fair or poor. The role that income plays in the elderly's self-assessment of their health status has become progressively more important, magni-fying the socioeconomic gap in well-being. This contradicts those (see Aday, Fleming, & Andersen, 1984) who assert that the gains made during the 1970s in access to better health and health care by the poor and disadvantaged have not been eroded by the fiscal austerity of the health care policies of the 1980s.

Living in the South (vs. living in the Midwest) or on a farm (vs. living in a small city or suburb of an SMSA) both have negative effects on perceived health status. Both of those effects become less impor-tant over time. The disadvantage of living in the South is reduced by more than one half during the course of the study, whereas the disadvantage of living on a farm dissipates entirely. When taken together, these results indicate that the once rather marked geographi-cal variations in perceived health status have declined considerably (see Aday & Eichhorn, 1972).

An examination of the effects of the cohort dummies and the intercepts facilitates an assessment of the net effects of age, period, and cohort on perceived health status. As indicated earlier, aging effects are reflected in the row comparisons of the cohort dummies. This reveals rather stable effects between the early 1970s and 1980s, followed by a consistent and significant decline between the early and mid-1980s. Indeed, with the exception of cohorts 2 through 4 (which exhibit some oscillation), the row comparisons yield equivalent (if not virtually isomorphic) coefficients in columns 1 through 3. No cohort, however, is significantly different from cohort 1 (the comparison group) or each other in column 4. When taken together, the consistent stability through the early 1980s and the consistent decline by the mid-1980s suggests the absence of any aging effects on perceived health status. Instead. they point to the presence of a period effect.

Comparing the intercepts yields additional support for such an interpretation. During the course of the study about a 25% reduction in the size of the intercept occurs. That is, all other things being equal, the perceived health status of elderly Americans suffered a significant decline over time. Moreover, most of that reduction occurs between the early and mid-1970s, and between the early and mid-1980s. Combined with the general absence of aging effects except for comparisons involving the mid-1980s, these changes in the intercepts are indicative of rather strong period effects.

Age-strata comparisons confirm this. When the coefficients for the cohort dummies (for cohorts 2 through 8) are compared within columns 1 through 3, age-graded differences occur 15 out of 18 times. These differences indicate that older age-groups view their health status as better than their younger counterparts. Although such comparisons involve both aging and cohort effects, the absence of any observed aging effects indicates that these age-strata differences must be the result of cohort effects. That is, all other things being equal, older cohorts view their health status more positively than do younger cohorts. This probably reflects the declining adherence to the more traditional and stoic acceptance of life and health hypothesized by Illich (1976) and to some extent documented by Elder (Elder, 1974, 1975; Elder & Liker, 1982), Haug and Lavin (1978, 1981, 1983), and Wolinsky and Wolinsky (1981).

Moreover, the absence of any significant age-strata comparisons in column 4 helps to clarify the nature of the period effect there. Conjointly, these data suggest that the period effect (i.e., the decline in perceived health status) observed for the mid-1980s wiped out the discriminating effects of the age-strata. That is, the mid-1980s period effect suppressed perceived health status to the point that cohort differences were no longer palpable. This implies that some historical change occurred in the mid-1980s that was so detrimental to the elderly as a class, that intraclass variations ceased being important. The most plausible historical change would have been the Medicare system's shift to the PPS and DRGs (see Fetter, Shin, Freeman, Avarill, & Thompson, 1980). The question of whether the negative impact and controversy surrounding PPS and DRGs was sufficient (in and of itself) to eliminate age-strata–based distinctions in the general well-being of the elderly, however, cannot be resolved with these data.

Table 5.2 contains the results of the regression-based cohort analysis of the degree of limited activity owing to health reasons. The results show that the predisposing and enabling characteristics explain 10.0% to 12.9% of the variance. Limited activity is positively related to experiencing widowhood, being black, living in the South or West (vs. living in the Midwest), and being a certain age. At the same time, limited activity is negatively related to being a woman, attaining education, being Hispanic, participating in the labor force, living alone, having income, having a telephone, living in the Northeast (vs. living in the Midwest), and living in the central city of an SMSA (vs. living in a smaller city or suburb of an SMSA). With the exception of living in the Northeast or in the central city of an SMSA, these relationships are replicated within each column of Table 5.2. Moreover, they are generally consistent with those reported in the literature (see Cornoni-Huntley, et al., 1985).

For most of the predisposing and enabling characteristics, significant changes in the magnitudes of the coefficients are observed over time. This includes being a woman, experiencing widowhood, attaining education, being black or Hispanic, living alone, having income, having a telephone, and living in the South, the West, or in the central city of an SMSA. Only the changes associated with income, however, constitute a clear pattern. Indeed, the variations in the coefficients for the other variables more closely approximate oscillations.

Income always produces a significant and negative effect. Individuals with greater family incomes are less likely to have activity limitations owing to health problems than those with lower family incomes. Over time, however, the negative effect of income becomes progressively more pronounced. Those increases are significant regardless of which columns are involved in the comparisons. During the course of the study period, the effect of income increases almost threefold. By the mid-1980s, every $10,000 increment in family income results in older Americans being 12% less likely to have activity limitations. Thus, as was the case for perceived health status, the socioeconomic

Table 5.2 Unstandardized Regression Coefficients (and Their Standard Errors) Obtained by Predicting Limited Activity Owing to Health Reasons, for All Cohorts Combined, by Survey Year*

Independent variables	Survey years 1972-73	1976-77	1980-81	1984-85
PREDISPOSING				
Demographic				
Sex	-.124 (.005)	-.125 (.005)	-.126 (.005)	-.054 (.006)
Widowhood	.030 (.007)	.045 (.007)	.039 (.008)	.039 (.008)
Social structure				
Education	-.011 (.001)	-.010 (.001)	-.012 (.001)	-.009 (.001)
Black	.039 (.009)	.040 (.010)	.038 (.010)	.019 (.009)
Hispanic	-.079 (.031)	-.117 (.017)	-.050 (.017)	-.039 (.017)
Labor force	-.241 (.006)	-.242 (.006)	-.241 (.006)	-.232 (.006)
Living alone	-.030 (.007)	-.059 (.008)	-.049 (.008)	-.027 (.008)
ENABLING				
Family				
Income	-.043 (.003)	-.063 (.003)	-.093 (.005)	-.120 (.006)
Telephone	-.028 (.009)	-.051 (.011)	-.045 (.013)	-.031 (.014)
Community				
Northeast		-.033 (.007)	-.029 (.007)	
South	.044 (.006)	.026 (.006)	.016 (.006)	.040 (.007)
West	.044 (.007)	.042 (.008)	.022 (.007)	.029 (.008)
Farm				
Central city	-.011 (.005)	-.013 (.005)	-.018 (.006)	
COHORT STRUCTURE				
Cohort 2		-.034 (.008)		-.041 (.010)
Cohort 3	-.021 (.007)	-.018 (.009)		-.034 (.011)
Cohort 4	-.022 (.008)		.039 (.011)	
Cohort 5	.020 (.009)		.088 (.013)	.087 (.017)
Cohort 6	.049 (.010)	.045 (.013)	.115 (.017)	.212 (.025)
Cohort 7	.077 (.012)	.117 (.017)	.177 (.026)	.202 (.050)
Cohort 8	.119 (.016)	.179 (.026)	.163 (.049)	.264 (.083)
Cohort 9	.202 (.022)		.018 (.007)	.073 (.007)
Intercept	.683 (.012)	.762 (.014)	.792 (.016)	.665 (.018)
R^2	.125	.123	.129	.100
N of Cases	41,093	36,230	35,588	32,348

*Coefficients not significantly different from 0 at the .05 probability level or beyond are omitted for clarity.

gap in limited activity continues to grow despite assertions to the contrary (see Aday et al., 1984).

Examining the cohort dummies and the intercepts facilitates an assessment of the net effects of age, period, and cohort. The row comparisons indicate a general pattern of aging effects for cohorts 4 through 8. As these cohorts age, their members are more likely to experience some activity limitations owing to health reasons. This is consistent with the extant literature (see Cornoni-Huntley et al., 1985) and reflects the physiological decline (and concomitant increase in limited activity) associated with age. What is not consistent is the absence of any consistent pattern of aging effects for cohorts 2 and 3. That may reflect a threshold effect, specifying that the onset of the increase in limited activity does not occur until the cohorts reach their mid- to late 60s.

At first glance, comparing the intercepts fails to yield a consistent pattern of period effects. The intercept obtained in the early 1970s is significantly smaller than that obtained in the mid-1970s. A comparison of the intercepts in columns 2 and 3 reveals the same pattern, although the difference is not significant. The intercept for the mid-1980s, however, is significantly smaller than that obtained in the early 1980s, or than that obtained in the mid-1970s. Thus, although a steady increase in the intercept occurs through the early 1980s, a sharp decline in it occurs by the mid-1980s.

The sharp decline in the intercept associated with the mid-1980s probably reflects the change in instrumentation regarding the limited activity question (see Chapter 3). It was in the mid-1980s that the National Center for Health Statistics (NCHS) modified the question in the HIS for those aged 70 or older. Rather than being asked if they had any limitations in their major activity (such as work), those older than 70 were asked if they had any limitations in their ability to care for themselves. Inasmuch as the latter requires greater physical limitations before abilities are jeopardized, the decline in the intercept (in the face of prior increases) is understandable. Indeed, it is likely that had no instrumentation change occurred, the intercepts for limited activity would have continued to indicate poorer health over time, just as the intercepts for perceived health did. Such a pattern is consistent with (but should not be taken as definitive support for) Fries's (1980) notion of the compression of morbidity.

Cohort differences can be found by making the age-strata comparisons within columns. In general, the coefficients for the cohort dummies indicate that limited activity increases from one age-group to the next for cohorts 4 through 8. This is similar to the pattern of aging effects reported earlier. Inasmuch as these age-strata comparisons involve both cohort and aging effects, and because aging effects have already been identified, these age-strata differences probably reflect aging and not cohort effects.

When taken together, the aging and cohort effects (or their absence) for the perceived health and limited activity measures are rather interesting. No aging effects were found for perceived health, but cohort effects were detected. In contrast, aging effects were found for limited activity, but cohort effects were not. This suggests that the elderly's more subjective assessments of their health status (i.e., perceived health) are relatively stable over their life course, but that their more objective assessments (i.e., whether they suffer from activity limitations because of health reasons) are not. This underscores prior observations and suggests that the elderly are more likely to discount responding to increasing levels of physical activity limitations because they are assumed to be part of the unavoidable circumstances of old age (see Ferraro, 1980; Wolinsky, Arnold, & Nallapati, 1988). Furthermore, it suggests that the more subjective health status assessments are subject to cohort succession-based changes, but that the more objective health status assessments are not. This also underscores prior observations and suggests that the perceived health status question reflects more of a global assessment (world view or perspective) that is enmeshed in the situational context of one's formative years (see Elder, 1974, 1975; Elder & Liker, 1982).

Use of Informal Health Services

Table 5.3 contains the results of the regression-based cohort analysis of the taking of restricted activity days. The results show that the predisposing, enabling, and need characteristics explain 11.1% to 14.2% of the variance. The taking of restricted activity days is positively related to being a woman, experiencing widowhood, being black, living alone, living in the South or West (vs. living in the Midwest), living in the central city of an SMSA (vs. living in a smaller city or suburb of an SMSA), and having limited activity because of health reasons. At the same time, the taking of restricted activity days is negatively related to educational attainment, labor force participation, life on a farm (vs. life in a small city or suburb of an SMSA), perceived health status, and age. For the most part, these effects are replicated within each column of Table 5.3 (the exceptions include widowhood, educational attainment, and income). These effects are also generally consistent with previous analyses of the taking of re-

Table 5.3 Unstandardized Regression Coefficients (and Their Standard Errors) Obtained by Predicting the Taking of Any Restricted Activity Days During Past Weeks, for All Cohorts Combined, by Survey Year*

Independent variables	Survey years			
	1972-73	1976-77	1980-81	1984-85
PREDISPOSING				
Demographic				
Sex	.018 (.004)	.025 (.004)	.029 (.004)	.009 (.004)
Widowhood	.013 (.005)			
Social structure				
Education	-.001 (.000)			
Black	.030 (.006)	.026 (.007)	.016 (.007)	.019 (.006)
Hispanic				
Labor force	-.024 (.004)	-.020 (.005)	-.014 (.005)	
Living alone	.018 (.005)	.029 (.006)	.025 (.006)	.017 (.005)
ENABLING				
Family				
Income			-.011 (.004)	
Telephone				
Community				
Northeast				
South	.015 (.004)	.009 (.005)		.017 (.005)
West	.012 (.005)	.026 (.006)	.039 (.006)	.028 (.005)
Farm		-.026 (.009)	-.020 (.010)	-.037 (.013)
Central City		.011 (.004)		.010 (.004)
NEED				
Limited activity	.138 (.004)	.162 (.004)	.170 (.004)	.132 (.004)
Perceived health	-.138 (.004)	-.142 (.005)	-.165 (.005)	-.153 (.005)
COHORT STRUCTURE				
Cohort 2	-.013 (.005)	-.024 (.006)		
Cohort 3	-.026 (.006)	-.019 (.006)	-.018 (.007)	
Cohort 4	-.028 (.006)	-.021 (.007)	-.020 (.008)	
Cohort 5	-.036 (.007)	-.032 (.008)	-.035 (.010)	
Cohort 6	-.043 (.008)	-.025 (.010)	-.041 (.013)	
Cohort 7	-.047 (.009)	-.032 (.013)	-.064 (.020)	
Cohort 8	-.032 (.012)			
Cohort 9	-.035 (.016)	.013 (.005)	.023 (.005)	.017 (.005)
Intercept	.215 (.010)	.197 (.011)	.201 (.013)	.175 (.013)
R^2	.111	.121	.142	.124
N of Cases	41,093	36,230	35,588	32,348

*Coefficients not significantly different from 0 at the .05 probability level or beyond are omitted for clarity.

stricted activity days, and as expected indicate that the need character-istics have the greatest salience (see Wolinsky et al., 1983).

Some significant and patterned changes in the magnitudes of the effects of five of the predisposing, enabling, and need characteristics occur over time. These involve being a woman, participating in the labor force, living in the West (vs. living in the Midwest), having limited activity, and perceived health status. The positive effect of being a woman on the taking of restricted activity days declines during the course of the study. Most of that decline occurs between columns 3 and 4. This may reflect a general change in gender role differentia-tion that did not become palpable among the elderly until the mid-1980s (see Krause, 1988). Confidence in this interpretation, how-ever, is limited given the absence of data from the late 1980s with which to establish such a trend.

The negative effect of labor-force participation consistently be-comes less important. Between the early 1970s and the early 1980s, the coefficient shrinks by some 40%. By the mid-1980s, the coeffi-cient is no longer significantly different from 0. One interpretation of these results is that the work environment for elderly individuals has progressively become more tolerable, allowing them greater opportu-nities to take restricted activity days without fear of retribution (see Chen, 1988; Robinson, Coberly, & Paul, 1985). Although plausible, that interpretation must remain speculative until better data are avail-able.

Between the early 1970s and the mid-1980s the effect of living in the West (vs. living in the Midwest) becomes significantly more important. Indeed, the coefficient more than doubles in magnitude. This may reflect the growing importance of the western region as a retirement haven. (Note that the effect of living in the South is rather consistent over time.) With increasing numbers of elderly individuals having better socioeconomic situations migrating from the harsher midwestern climates to more temperate ones in the West, those migrating elderly may have greater opportunities to take restricted activity days. That is, the increasing salience of living in the West may be indicative of a favorable in-migration stream that is not captured by the socioeconomic status measures already in the model (see Longino & Soldo, 1987).

The changes in the effects of the health status measures are some-what puzzling. Limited activity's positive effect increases from the early 1970s through the early 1980s but almost returns to its original level by the mid-1980s. Similarly, the negative effect of perceived health status increases from the early 1970s through the early 1980s, and then significantly declines by the mid-1980s. That mid-1980s effect, however, remains significantly greater than its counterpart from the early 1970s. Taken together, the changes in the effects of the health status measures suggest statistical interaction involving the mid-1980s. That is, some historical event must have occurred that was sufficient to nullify (or reverse) the trend of increasing magnitudes of effect. It is plausible that this is related to the fiscal austerity that the elderly faced during the Reagan administration (see Mechanic, 1985). That is, when faced with increasingly limited resources and access to health care, elderly individuals as a class were forced to raise their tolerance thresholds for illnesses before turning to informal health services. These data, however, are not sufficient to corroborate such an effect.

An assessment of the net effects of age, period, and cohort on the taking of restricted activity days is facilitated by examining the effects of the cohort dummies and the intercepts. The row comparisons reveal no consistent patterns of change in the cohort dummies. Thus, no aging effects occur. Comparing the intercepts does reveal a period effect, but only when the coefficients from the early 1970s and the mid-1980s are involved. That comparison reflects a modest decline in the taking of restricted activity days, all other things being equal. Finally, the age-strata comparisons within columns indicate that, more often than not, older cohorts take fewer restricted activity days. This is consistent with the view that those older cohorts are more likely to exhibit stoic health behavior and greater tolerance of health problems than their younger counterparts (see Elder, 1974, 1975; Elder & Liker, 1982). The magnitude of those cohort differences, however, is modest and is usually not manifest in successive comparisons. Thus, when taken together, these comparisons suggest the absence of any appreciable age, period, or cohort effects on the taking of restricted activity days.

Table 5.4 contains the results of the regression-based cohort analysis of the taking of bed disability days. The results show that from 10.0% to 12.4% of the variance can be explained. The taking of bed disability days is positively related to being a woman, experiencing widowhood, being black, being Hispanic, living in the South or West (vs. living in the Midwest), living in the central city of an SMSA (vs. living in a smaller city or suburb of an SMSA), and having limited activity because of health reasons. At the same time, the taking of bed disability days is negatively related to labor-force participation, possession of a telephone, life on a farm (vs. life in a small city or suburb of an SMSA), perceived health status, and age. These results are

Table 5.4 Unstandardized Regression Coefficients (and Their Standard Errors) Obtained by Predicting the Taking of Bed Disability Days During Past Weeks, for All Cohorts Combined, by Survey Year*

Independent variables	Survey years			
	1972-73	1976-77	1980-81	1984-85
PREDISPOSING				
Demographic				
Sex		.015 (.003)	.015 (.003)	
Widowhood	.015 (.004)			
Social structure				
Education				
Black	.015 (.005)		.020 (.005)	.010 (.005)
Hispanic	.046 (.016)			.039 (.009)
Labor force	-.015 (.003)	-.012 (.003)		-.012 (.003)
Living alone				
ENABLING				
Family				
Income				
Telephone		-.028 (.006)	-.015 (.007)	-.019 (.008)
Community				
Northeast				
South	.009 (.003)			
West			.010 (.004)	.010 (.004)
Farm	-.014 (.005)		-.018 (.007)	-.029 (.010)
Central city	.011 (.003)	.008 (.003)		.008 (.003)
NEED				
Limited activity	.049 (.003)	.054 (.003)	.058 (.003)	.070 (.003)
Perceived health	-.078 (.003)	-.083 (.003)	-.075 (.003)	-.097 (.003)
COHORT STRUCTURE				
Cohort 2		-.009 (.004)		
Cohort 3	-.017 (.004)	-.014 (.005)		
Cohort 4	-.020 (.004)	-.011 (.005)		
Cohort 5	-.023 (.005)			
Cohort 6	-.022 (.005)			
Cohort 7	-.023 (.007)			
Cohort 8				
Cohort 9			.014 (.004)	.010 (.004)
Intercept	.105 (.007)	.124 (.008)	.100 (.009)	.115 (.010)
R^2	.050	.051	.051	.078
N of Cases	41,093	36,230	35,588	32,348

*Coefficients not significantly different from 0 at the .05 probability level or beyond are omitted for clarity.

generally consistent with those obtained in prior studies, and as expected indicate that the biggest predictors of taking bed disability days are the health-status measures (see Wolinsky et al., 1983).

In contrast to the patterns observed in the previous tables, many of the effects manifest for the predisposing, enabling, and need characteristics shown in Table 5.4 are not replicated in all of the columns. Only the effects of being black, participating in the labor force, having a telephone, living on a farm or in the central city of an SMSA (vs. living in a smaller city or suburb of an SMSA), having limited activity, and having perceived health produce significant effects in at least three columns. It is only for the health status measures that the effects are replicated in all four columns. Moreover, the magnitude of the observed effects is not large. In part this results from the attenuation that occurs when a relatively rare event (like the taking of bed disability days in the past 2 weeks) is predicted.

Nonetheless, the effects of the predisposing, enabling, and need characteristics shown in Table 5.4 are rather stable. That is, when an effect is detected, it neither exhibits a trend nor oscillates across the columns. The exceptions here are the effects of the health status measures. Both of them register significant increases in magnitude from the early 1970s to the mid-1980s. Those increases, however, occur principally between the third and fourth columns. This suggests an interaction involving that particular period (i.e., the mid-1980s), which is similar to that observed in Table 5.3 for the taking of restricted activity days. Again, it is plausible that these increases result from the negative impact of the fiscal austerity associated with the health care policies of the 1980s (see Mechanic, 1985).

Examining the effects of the cohort dummies and the intercepts facilitates an assessment of the net effects of age, period, and cohort on the taking of bed disability days. The row comparisons reveal no meaningful aging effects on the coefficients for the cohort dummies. Although some of the cohort dummies produced significant effects in the early 1970s, those effects were marginal and not reproduced over time. Similarly, a comparison of the intercepts indicates that although some oscillation occurs, no consistent trend is observed. Finally, no significant age-strata differences are found within the columns. Thus, when taken taken together, these comparisons suggest that there are no net age, period, or cohort effects on the taking of bed disability days. This is entirely consistent with the results observed for the taking of restricted activity days. Accordingly, it appears that for the most part, the use of informal health services is not subject to net age, period, or cohort effects.

Use of Formal Health Services

Dentists' Services

Table 5.5 contains the results of the regression-based cohort analysis of the dental contact measure. The results show that 13.9% to 15.3% of the variance can be explained. Dental contact rates are positively related to being a woman, attaining education, living alone, having income, having a telephone, living anywhere except the Midwest, living in the central city of an SMSA (vs. living in a smaller city or suburb of an SMSA), and having perceived health. At the same time, dental contact rates are negatively related to widowhood, life on a farm (vs. life in a small city or suburb of an SMSA), limited activity, and age. These results are generally reproduced within each column of Table 5.5. They are also consistent with the results of previous studies (see Wolinsky & Arnold, 1988).

Four variables are among the predisposing, enabling, and need characteristics for which significant and patterned changes in the magnitude of the coefficients occur. These are income, having a telephone, living in the South (vs. living in the Midwest), and living in the central city of an SMSA (vs. living in a smaller city or suburb of an SMSA). The income effect produces the most striking changes. Between the early 1970s and the early 1980s, the coefficient for income nearly doubles. This indicates that income progressively becomes a more important barrier between the elderly and the dental services that they need. Accordingly, considerable and expanding inequality appears to exist with respect to the oral health care of aged Americans (see Wolinsky & Arnold, 1989).

The effect of having a telephone also increases over time. Having a telephone in the early 1980s makes one significantly more likely to have seen a dentist than it did in the early 1970s. The magnitude of that increase is approximately 50%. This likely represents an increased reliance of dentists on telephone follow-ups to remind elderly (and for that matter, nonelderly) patients of their annual checkups. Such action would be consistent with the more competitive environment facing dentists in the 1980s (see Department of Health and Human Services, 1982). This interpretation, however, cannot be further assessed with these data.

The effects of living in the South (vs. living in the Midwest) or in the central city of an SMSA (vs. living in a smaller city or suburb of an SMSA) both decline over time. Indeed, although both residence measures yield consistent and significant effects in the 1970s, those effects fully dissipate by the early 1980s. This most likely reflects the

Table 5.5 Unstandardized Regression Coefficients (and Their Standard Errors) Obtained by Predicting Dental Contact During the Past Year, for All Cohorts Combined, by Survey Year*

Independent variables	Survey years		
	1972-73	1976-77	1980-81
PREDISPOSING			
Demographic			
Sex	.040 (.005)	.042 (.005)	.035 (.005)
Widowhood	-.063 (.007)	-.072 (.008)	-.060 (.008)
Social structure			
Education	.024 (.001)	.026 (.001)	.028 (.001)
Black		-.025 (.010)	
Hispanic			.065 (.017)
Labor force			
Living alone	.088 (.007)	.098 (.008)	.088 (.008)
ENABLING			
Family			
Income	.078 (.003)	.101 (.003)	.142 (.005)
Telephone	.058 (.009)	.094 (.011)	.088 (.013)
Community			
Northeast	.040 (.006)	.027 (.007)	.031 (.007)
South	.029 (.006)	.031 (.006)	
West	.060 (.007)	.065 (.008)	.045 (.008)
Farm	-.025 (.010)		-.037 (.014)
Central city	.023 (.005)	.015 (.005)	
NEED			
Limited activity		-.015 (.006)	-.012 (.006)
Perceived health	.032 (.006)	.040 (.006)	.039 (.006)
COHORT STRUCTURE			
Cohort 2	-.022 (.007)		-.026 (.009)
Cohort 3	-.035 (.008)	-.048 (.009)	-.034 (.009)
Cohort 4	-.061 (.008)	-.062 (.009)	-.059 (.011)
Cohort 5	-.089 (.009)	-.094 (.011)	-.092 (.013)
Cohort 6	-.119 (.010)	-.113 (.013)	-.154 (.017)
Cohort 7	-.152 (.012)	-.161 (.017)	-.188 (.026)
Cohort 8	-.163 (.017)	-.149 (.027)	-.210 (.049)
Cohort 9	-.203 (.022)		.020 (.007)
Intercept		-.077 (.015)	-.103 (.017)
R^2	.139	.150	.153
N of Cases	41,093	36,230	35,588

*Coefficients not significantly different from 0 at the .05 probability level or beyond are omitted for clarity.

effective market redistribution of dentists brought about by their increasing supply and resultant competition (see Department of Health and Human Services, 1982). This interpretation is further supported by the (albeit not statistically significant) trend toward greater geographical equity exhibited in the effects for the other residential location variables.

The net effects of age, period, and cohort on dental contact rates are revealed by an examination of the effects of the cohort dummies and the intercepts. The row comparisons of the coefficients for the cohort dummies indicate that no consistent aging effects occur. Indeed, the coefficients for cohorts 2 through 5 are virtually isomorphic across rows. Although changes do occur for cohorts 6 through 8, the bulk of these changes occur between the mid-1970s and the early 1980s. This suggests an interaction between age and period but only for the oldest-old. As such, it probably reflects the fact that double-digit inflation occurred during this period. It likely affected the oldest-old more than their younger counterparts, because the oldest-old's general economic wealth is substantially lower (see Atkins, 1985), and their assets are disproportionately less liquid (see Torrey, 1985).

A comparison of the intercepts shows no significant changes, indicating that no period effects exist. In contrast, the age-strata comparisons within columns yield consistent (with one exception) increases across age-groups. That is, the older the cohort, the lower the dental contact rate. When taken together, then, these data indicate that the age-related changes observed in Table 5.5 are a result of cohort succession. Younger cohorts having higher dental contact rates are replacing older cohorts having lower dental contact rates (see Wolinsky & Arnold, 1989). If this pattern of cohort succession continues, then aggregate dental contact rates will continue to increase without any change occurring in the oral health behavior of individual older Americans.

The identification of cohort succession effects on dental contact rates is intuitively pleasing for three reasons. First, it is consistent with the view that oral health behavior is a relatively stable trait among adults (see Kiyak, 1987). Second, oral health practices are an excellent example of personal behaviors for which the pattern formation at early ages is highly influenced by example and cues (see Kegeles, 1963). Therefore, as standards for oral health care, hygiene, and appearance change over time, successive birth cohorts are socialized to dissimilar expectations. Third, and as indicated in Chapter 3, the use of dentists' services is the most discretionary of the formal health services (see Andersen, 1968; Andersen & Newman, 1973). As such, it is likely to be the most sensitive to normative changes.

Physicians' Services

Table 5.6 contains the results of the regression-based cohort analysis of the physician contact measure. The results indicate that from 5.4% to 6.5% of the variance can be explained. Having contacted a physician during the past 12 months is positively related to being a woman, attaining education, living alone, having income, having a telephone, living in the Northeast (vs. living in the Midwest, but only in the mid-1980s), having limited activity owing to health reasons, and being a certain age. At the same time, having contacted a physician is negatively related to participating in the labor force (but only in the mid-1980s), living on a farm (vs. living in a small city or suburb of an SMSA, but only in the mid-1970s and early 1980s), and perceived health status. Except for the parenthetical entries noted earlier, these effects are registered for each column of Table 5.6. Moreover, these results are consistent with the extant literature on physician contact rates among the elderly. They indicate that the most powerful predictors are the health status measures (see Wolinsky & Arnold, 1988).

Four variables are among the predisposing, enabling, and need characteristics whose effects reflect significant and patterned changes over time. These are status as a woman, income, limited activity, and perceived health status. The positive effect of being a woman diminishes during the course of the study. That decline, however, is rather modest. Indeed, although a monotonic trend exists throughout, the only comparison that yields significant differences occurs when the coefficient for the early 1970s is compared with that from the mid-1980s. Even then, the disparate confidence intervals are not far apart. Thus, these data suggest only a rather gradual narrowing of the gender gap in physician contact rates consistent with the declining significance of gender in health behavior (see Verbrugge, 1985).

The positive effect of income increases in magnitude with each successive comparison. In the early 1970s its effect was such that every $10,000 increment resulted in an increased probability of physician contact of .03. By the mid-1980s, that increased proability had more than doubled to .067. Thus, income progressively became a more important barrier between the elderly and the physicians' services that they need. Moreover, although the increasing effect of

Table 5.6 Unstandardized Regression Coefficients (and Their Standard Errors) Obtained by Predicting Physici Contact During the Past Year, for All Cohorts Combined, by Survey Year*

Independent	Survey years			
variables	1972-73	1976-77	1980-81	1984-85
PREDISPOSING				
Demographic				
Sex	.059 (.005)	.055 (.005)	.048 (.005)	.046 (.005)
Widowhood				
Social structure				
Education	.006 (.001)	.005 (.001)	.005 (.001)	.004 (.001)
Black				
Hispanic				
Labor force				-.027 (.005)
Living alone	.022 (.007)	.029 (.007)	.023 (.007)	.029 (.007)
ENABLING				
Family				
Income	.031 (.002)	.038 (.003)	.044 (.004)	.067 (.005)
Telephone	.133 (.008)	.109 (.010)	.112 (.012)	.113 (.012)
Community				
Northeast				.013 (.006)
South				
West				
Farm		-.028 (.011)	-.030 (.012)	
Central city				
NEED				
Limited activity	.148 (.005)	.138 (.005)	.145 (.005)	.127 (.005)
Perceived health	-.104 (.005)	-.082 (.005)	-.087 (.006)	-.084 (.006)
COHORT STRUCTURE				
Cohort 2			.036 (.008)	.027 (.008)
Cohort 3	.015 (.007)	.039 (.008)	.050 (.008)	.037 (.009)
Cohort 4	.025 (.008)	.046 (.008)	.055 (.010)	.047 (.011)
Cohort 5	.039 (.008)	.031 (.009)	.044 (.012)	.029 (.015)
Cohort 6	.033 (.010)	.029 (.011)	.030 (.015)	
Cohort 7	.028 (.011)			
Cohort 8	.034 (.016)			
Cohort 9				-.037 (.006)
Intercept	.479 (.012)	.529 (.013)	.520 (.015)	.564 (.016)
R^2	.065	.054	.056	.058
N of Cases	41,093	36,230	35,588	32,348

*Coefficients not significantly different from 0 at the .05 probability level or beyond are omitted for clarity.

income is significant regardless of which comparison is made, that effect increases most between the early and mid-1980s. This was precisely the time during which fiscal austerity programs introduced at the federal level (i.e., cutbacks in Medicare funding) were said to place the elderly at greatest jeopardy (see Mechanic, 1985).

The effects of limited activity and perceived health status also change over time. These changes, however, are limited to one successive comparison each. For limited activity, the comparison that yields a significant difference in the coefficients involves the early and mid-1980s. During this period, a significant reduction in the effect of limited activity occurs. This probably reflects the instrumentation change in the HISs introduced by the NCHS at that time. In contrast, the only comparison that yields a significant change in the coefficient for perceived health status involves the early to mid-1970s. During this period a significant reduction of the effect occurs. It is impossible, however, to determine whether this represents the end of a steady trend without additional columns of data (prior to the 1970s).

Comparing the effects of the cohort dummies and the intercepts facilitates an assessment of the net effects of age, period, and cohort. The row comparisons of these coefficients for the dummy variables indicate that no consistent aging effects occur. Indeed, of the 12 possible successive comparisons, only 2 yield significant differences. Thus, no meaningful age-related changes occur. Similarly, age-strata comparisons within columns also fail to yield any significant differences. This indicates the absence of any cohort-related changes.

A comparison of the intercepts, however, does yield significant period effects. Here, palpable increases occur between the early and mid-1970s, and between the early and mid-1980s. During the course of the study, physician contact rates increased by about 8%. This is consistent with previously published reports (see Havlik, et al., 1987) and reflects the increase in the relative supply of physicians (see Department of Health and Human Services, 1982).

Table 5.7 contains the results of the regression-based cohort analysis of the number of physician visits during the past year, among those with at least one visit. The results show that from 14.9% to 17.5% of the variance can be explained. The volume of physician visits is positively related to being a woman, experiencing widowhood, being black, being Hispanic, living alone, having income, having a telephone, living in the Northeast or West (vs. living in the Midwest), living in the central city of an SMSA (vs. living in a smaller city or suburb of an SMSA), and having limited activity. At the same time, the volume of physician visits is negatively related to educational

Table 5.7 Unstandardized Regression Coefficients (and Their Standard Errors) Obtained by Predicting Number of Physician Visits During Past Year (Among Those With Visits), for All Cohorts Combined, by Survey Year*

Independent	Survey years			
variables	1972-73	1976-77	1980-81	1984-85
PREDISPOSING				
Demographic				
Sex	.286 (.050)	.320 (.050)	.151 (.048)	.140 (.050)
Widowhood	.211 (.067)		.169 (.068)	
Social structure				
Education	-.025 (.007)	-.025 (.007)		
Black		.389 (.089)	.574 (.088)	.304 (.084)
Hispanic			.698 (.153)	.411 (.157)
Labor force	-.577 (.058)	-.479 (.059)	-.493 (.057)	-.414 (.059)
Living alone		.268 (.072)	.284 (.070)	.301 (.071)
ENABLING				
Family				
Income	.059 (.025)			
Telephone		.403 (.109)	.260 (.126)	.297 (.139)
Community				
Northeast	.372 (.061)	.297 (.063)		.283 (.065)
South	-.314 (.059)	-.184 (.059)	-.326 (.058)	-.250 (.061)
West	.251 (.070)	.160 (.070)	.182 (.068)	.308 (.070)
Farm		-.268 (.117)		
Central city	.229 (.049)	.224 (.050)	.171 (.050)	.194 (.052)
NEED				
Limited activity	1.762 (.053)	1.889 (.053)	1.641 (.051)	1.921 (.054)
Perceived health	-1.813 (.055)	-1.662 (.056)	-1.854 (.055)	-1.963 (.057)
COHORT STRUCTURE				
Cohort 2				
Cohort 3				.224 (.096)
Cohort 4				
Cohort 5				-.297 (.148)
Cohort 6				-.425 (.213)
Cohort 7	-.258 (.120)		-.471 (.232)	
Cohort 8		-.593 (.249)		
Cohort 9	-.604 (.219)	.183 (.069)		
Intercept	5.678 (.133)	5.000 (.147)	4.953 (.160)	4.891 (.172)
R^2	.149	.152	.154	.175
N of Cases	30,334	28,279	27,573	25,762

*Coefficients not significantly different from 0 at the .05 probability level or beyond are omitted for clarity.

attainment, labor-force participation, life in the South (vs. life in the Midwest), life on a farm (vs. life in a small city or suburb of an SMSA), perceived health status, and age. Of these effects, those for widowhood, educational attainment, a Hispanic background, income, and life on a farm are not consistently reproduced across the columns (i.e., they appear only once or twice). Nonetheless, these results are generally consistent with those reported in the extant literature and indicate that the most salient predictors of the volume of physician use are the need characteristics (see Wolinsky & Coe, 1984).

Significant changes occur in the magnitudes of the coefficients for four of the predisposing, enabling, and need characteristics. These are status as a woman, labor-force participation, life in the South (vs. life in the Midwest), and limited activity owing to health reasons. The positive effect of being a woman declines by about 50% over time. In the early 1970s the gender gap was about 0.29 visits. By the mid-1980s that gap had narrowed to 0.14 visits. Although most of that decline occurred between the mid-1970s and the early 1980s, a modest yet significant decline also occurred between the early and mid-1980s. This moderate decline in the gender gap is consistent with the extant literature (see Verbrugge, 1985).

The negative effect of labor-force participation also declines over time. That decline, however, is rather gradual. It is only palpable when the coefficient from the early 1970s is compared with that from the mid-1980s. Indeed, no significant changes are detected in any successive comparison. Moreover, the change only constitutes about a 25% decrement. Thus, the impact of labor-force participation is only modestly diminished and does not appear to reflect an important trend.

Living in the South (vs. living in the Midwest) produces relatively stable negative effects, with one exception. The effect for the mid-1970s is significantly less than that for either the early 1970s or the early 1980s. Even for that difference, however, the coefficients are only marginally outside of each other's confidence intervals. Accordingly, this lone exception is more indicative of fluctuation than it is of interpretable trend.

The effect of limited activity oscillates over time. Between the early and mid-1970s the effect of limited activity becomes significantly but modestly stronger. In contrast, between the mid-1970s and the early 1980s the effect of limited activity becomes significantly but modestly weaker. Finally, between the early and mid-1980s the effect of limited activity becomes significantly but modestly stronger once again. During the course of the study, the effect of limited activity experiences a significant but modest increase in its magnitude. Such a pattern is more indicative of fluctuation than of a meaningful trend, especially given the instrumentation changes that occur in the mid-1980s.

Examining the effects of the cohort dummies and the intercepts facilitates an assessment of the net effect of age, period, and cohort on the volume of physician visits. The row comparisons of the cohort dummies reveal an interesting two-part pattern. First, most of the cells of the table do not contain significant coefficients. This means that, all other things being equal, few age differences exist in the volume of physician visits. The second part of the pattern is that for cohorts 5 through 8, five of the coefficients are significant, and all of them are negative. Thus, when the older cohorts differ from the younger ones, the older cohorts actually have fewer visits to physicians.

This lower level of physician use among the older cohorts, however, does not represent an aging effect. The reason is that the pattern involves comparisons within columns (i.e., age-strata effects) rather than across rows (i.e., aging effects). Accordingly, these data suggest that a modest cohort effect exists such that the older cohorts have annual rates of physician use modestly lower than their younger counterparts. Accordingly, these data do not support the inverse J-curve identified by the traditional cohort analysis in Chapter 4 (see Wolinsky, Mosely, & Coe, 1986; Wolinsky et al., 1988). Instead, they are more consistent with the recent report of Shapiro and Tate (1989), whose panel analysis also indicates modest cohort effects in the absence of aging effects.

The comparison of the intercepts indicates that some period effects have occurred. Between the early and mid-1970s, the intercept declines by about two thirds of a physician visit. From the mid-1970s through the mid-1980s, however, the intercept remains relatively stable. When taken together, this suggests that the volume of physician visits was significantly reduced between the early and mid-1970s, but that since that time no further palpable changes have occurred. This is generally consistent with the results of the traditional cohort analysis reported in Chapter 4.

When taken together, the data in Tables 5.6 and 5.7 clarify the relationship between age and the use of physician services among older adults. No aging effects are detected, either for physician contact or for the annual number of physician visits (among those with visits). In contrast, period effects are detected for both measures. On the one hand, a significant increase occurs in physician contact rates during the study period. Conversely, a decline of about two thirds of a visit in the volume of physician visits occurs in the mid-1970s, with the reduced level remaining stable thereafter. Although these period effects may seem contradictory, they reflect the general increase in access to medical care (i.e., greater physician contact rates) coupled with increasing efforts at containing health care costs (i.e., reduced annual rates of physician use). Finally, these data reveal some modest cohort effects on the volume of physician use. Older cohorts appear to consume about one fourth to one half of a visit less than their younger counterparts.

Hospitals' Services

Table 5.8 contains the results of the regression-based cohort analysis of the hospital contact measure. The results show that from 5.6% to 7.4% of the variance can be explained. Having been hospitalized during the past 12 months is positively related to widowhood (but only in the mid-1980s), educational attainment (but only in the 1970s), life alone (but only in the early 1980s), income, possession of a telephone, limited activity, and age. At the same time, having been hospitalized is negatively related to being a woman, being black, being Hispanic (but only in the early 1980s), participating in the labor force, living in the Northeast or West (vs. living in the Midwest), living in the South (vs. living in the Midwest, but only during the early 1970s), living on a farm (vs. living in a small city or suburb of an SMSA, but only in the mid-1970s), living in the central city of an SMSA (vs. living in a smaller city or suburb of an SMSA, but only during the mid-1970s and early 1980s), and perceived health status. These relationships are generally consistent with those reported in the extant literature and indicate that the most salient predictors of hospitalization are the health-status measures (see Wolinsky & Coe, 1984).

The effects of five of the predisposing, enabling, and need characteristics exhibit significant changes over time. These are the effects of life as a black, labor-force participation, income, limited activity owing to health reasons, and perceived health status. The changes in the effects of life as a black and labor-force participation, however, do not reflect any consistent trend. Moreover, those changes involve only one significant comparison (the mid-1970s with the early 1980s for the effect of life as a black, and the mid-1970s with the mid-1980s for the effect of labor-force participation). Furthermore, for both variables the coefficients obtained at the beginning and the end of the study period are equivalent. Accordingly, these isolated changes should not be considered indicative of meaningful structural change in the demand for hospital contact.

Table 5.8 Unstandardized Regression Coefficients (and Their Standard Errors) Obtained by Predicting Hospital Contact During Past Year, for All Cohorts Combined, by Survey Year*

Independent	Survey years			
variables	1972-73	1976-77	1980-81	1984-85
PREDISPOSING				
Demographic				
Sex	-.021 (.004)	-.018 (.004)	-.019 (.004)	-.025 (.004)
Widowhood				.018 (.006)
Social structure				
Education	.002 (.001)	.001 (.001)		
Black	-.036 (.007)	-.040 (.008)	-.019 (.008)	-.034 (.007)
Hispanic			-.033 (.013)	
Labor force	-.026 (.004)	-.018 (.005)	-.021 (.005)	-.030 (.005)
Living alone			.015 (.006)	
ENABLING				
Family				
Income	.007 (.002)	.007 (.003)	.019 (.004)	.019 (.005)
Telephone	.034 (.007)	.034 (.009)	.022 (.010)	
Community				
Northeast	-.021 (.005)	-.020 (.005)	-.020 (.005)	-.017 (.006)
South	-.011 (.005)			
West		-.021 (.006)	-.025 (.006)	-.02 (.006)
Farm		-.025 (.010)		
Central city		-.009 (.004)	-.009 (.004)	
NEED				
Limited activity	.100 (.004)	.113 (.005)	.111 (.005)	.112 (.005)
Perceived health	-.098 (.004)	-.098 (.005)	-.103 (.005)	-.117 (.005)
COHORT STRUCTURE				
Cohort 2		.015 (.006)		.030 (.008)
Cohort 3		.028 (.007)	.030 (.007)	.058 (.009)
Cohort 4		.027 (.007)	.030 (.008)	.040 (.010)
Cohort 5	.025 (.007)	.041 (.008)	.037 (.010)	.050 (.013)
Cohort 6	.033 (.008)	.055 (.010)	.044 (.013)	.057 (.019)
Cohort 7	.023 (.009)	.052 (.013)		
Cohort 8	.029 (.013)			
Cohort 9				-.012 (.006)
Intercept	.147 (.010)	.145 (.012)	.156 (.013)	.188 (.014)
R^2	.056	.060	.062	.074
N of Cases	41,093	36,230	35,588	32,348

*Coefficients not significantly different from 0 at the .05 probability level or beyond are omitted for clarity.

In contrast, the change in the effect of income is quite patterned. The coefficients obtained in the 1970s are identical. Similarly, the coefficients obtained in the 1980s are also identical, but they are nearly three times as large as their 1970s counterparts. Thus, the financial barrier to hospitalization that family income represents became larger during the decade of the 1980s. This is consistent with the view that the economic downturn and fiscal austerity of the 1980s disenfranchised many individuals from the health care delivery system (see Berki et al., 1985; Mechanic, 1985).

The changes in the effects of limited activity and perceived health are rather similar. Both increase in magnitude over time by about 12% to 14%. Moreover, both changes fundamentally involve only one successive comparison. For limited activity the change occurs between the early and mid-1970s. In contrast, the change for perceived health occurs between the early and mid-1980s. These changes indicate that health status, whether more objectively (i.e., limited activity) or subjectively (i.e., perceived health) measured, has become even more important in predicting hospital contact. No consistent trends, however, can be identified.

The net effects of age, period, and cohort on hospital contact are reflected in the cohort dummies and the intercepts. Comparing the effects for the cohort dummies across the rows fails to indicate any consistent pattern of aging effects. Indeed, even when the comparisons involve the most time-distant coefficients, only one significant difference is found (involving cohort 3). Similarly, only two age-strata differences are found when the coefficients are successively compared within columns. When taken together, the row and column comparisons of the cohort dummies indicate that neither aging nor cohort effects are occurring with respect to hospital contact.

A comparison of the intercepts, however, does reveal a significant period effect. The intercept obtained in the mid-1980s is significantly greater than those obtained for the previous periods, all of which are equivalent. This indicates that, all other things being equal, the likelihood of having been hospitalized in the past 12 months increased significantly between the early and mid-1980s. This is exactly the period during which Medicare switched to the PPS system and its associated DRGs. As indicated in Chapter 4, some critics of this system suspect that it will result in raising the hospital admission rate at the same time that it lowers the average length of stay (see Wolinsky, 1988). These results (which are a partial analogue of admission rates) are entirely consistent with those suspicions.

Table 5.9 contains the results of the regression-based cohort analysis of the number of hospital episodes that occurred during the past 12 months, among those with at least one episode. The results show that from 4.3% to 5.6% of the variance can be explained. The number of hospital episodes is positively related to widowhood and educational attainment (but only in the early 1970s) and limited activity. At the same time, the number of hospital episodes is negatively related to being a woman, being black (but only in the early 1980s), participating in the labor force, living alone (but only in the early 1970s), living outside of the midwest, living in the central city of an SMSA (vs. living in a smaller city or suburb of an SMSA), and perceived health status. In general, these results are consistent with those reported in the extant literature (see Wolinsky & Coe, 1984).

The effects of only two of the predisposing, enabling, and need characteristics significantly change over time. These are the effects of being a woman and perceived health status. The change in the effect of being a woman involves comparing the coefficient from the mid-1970s with that from the mid-1980s. These coefficients marginally fall outside of each other's confidence intervals, indicating a modest increase in the gender gap. No significant difference exists, however, between the coefficient obtained in the early 1970s and that obtained in the mid-1980s. Thus, the one successive comparison described earlier most likely reflects a fluctuation rather than any patterned change.

A different story is told by the changes in the effect of perceived health. The coefficients obtained in the 1970s are equivalent, as are the coefficients obtained in the 1980s. Both of the 1970s coefficients are significantly greater than each of the 1980s coefficients. The magnitude of those differences, however, is rather marginal. Nonetheless, this indicates that a significant increase occurred in the role of perceived health in determining the number of hospital episodes in the 1980s. It could be yet another reflection of the fiscal austerity that the elderly faced during the Reagan administration (see Mechanic, 1985).

Comparing the effects of the cohort dummies and the intercepts facilitates an assessment of the net effects of aging, period, and cohort. None of the cohort dummies produced significant coefficients. Therefore, neither aging nor cohort effects exist. A comparison of the intercepts, however, does reveal a modest period effect. The intercept obtained in the early 1970s is significantly less than those obtained subsequently. The intercepts obtained from the mid-1970s to the mid-1980s are all equivalent. This indicates that, all other things being equal, an increase occurred in the number of hospital episodes in the early 1970s, but that since then no significant changes have occurred.

Table 5.9 Unstandardized Regression Coefficients (and Their Standard Errors) Obtained by Predicting Number of Hospital Episodes During Past Year (Among Those With Episodes), for All Cohorts Combined, by Survey Year*

Independent variables	Survey years			
	1972-73	1976-77	1980-81	1984-85
PREDISPOSING				
Demographic				
Sex	-.065 (.022)	-.050 (.022)		-.112 (.027)
Widowhood	.062 (.030)			
Social structure				
Education	.007 (.003)			
Black			-.162 (.046)	
Hispanic				
Labor force	-.105 (.028)	-.091 (.029)	-.084 (.032)	
Living alone	-.065 (.031)			
ENABLING				
Family				
Income				
Telephone				
Community				
Northeast	-.079 (.028)		-.106 (.033)	-.072 (.036)
South	-.054 (.026)			-.092 (.032)
West			-.078 (.036)	-.147 (.039)
Farm				
Central city			-.094 (.026)	-.084 (.028)
NEED				
Limited activity	.166 (.023)	.150 (.024)	.174 (.027)	.201 (.029)
Perceived health	-.181 (.023)	-.184 (.024)	-.238 (.026)	-.279 (.029)
COHORT STRUCTURE				
Cohort 2				
Cohort 3				
Cohort 4				
Cohort 5				
Cohort 6				
Cohort 7				
Cohort 8				
Cohort 9				
Intercept	1.260 (.058)	1.443 (.065)	1.441 (.077)	1.597 (.087)
R^2	.050	.043	.054	.056
N of Cases	6,218	5,868	5,646	5,297

*Coefficients not significantly different from 0 at the .05 probability level or beyond are omitted for clarity.

Accordingly, these data do not support the suspicion that Medicare's shift to the PPS system has increased the number of hospitalizations among those having at least one such episode (see Wolinsky, 1988).

Table 5.10 contains the results of the regression-based cohort analysis of the number of nights spent in the hospital during the past 12 months, among those with hospital episodes. The results show that from 8.9% to 10.0% of the variance can be explained. The number of nights spent in the hospital is positively related to experiencing widowhood (but only in the 1970s), being black (but only in the 1970s), living in the Northeast (vs. living in the Midwest), living in the central city of an SMSA (vs. living in a smaller city or suburb of an SMSA, but only in the early 1970s and mid-1980s), having limited activity, and being a certain age. At the same time, the number of nights spent in the hospital is negatively related to being a woman (but not in the early 1980s), participating in the labor force, living in the South (vs. living in the Midwest, but not in the early 1970s or the early 1980s), living on a farm (vs. living in a small city or suburb of an SMSA, but not in the mid-1970s or mid-1980s), and perceived health status. These results are generally consistent with those reported in the extant literature (see Wolinsky & Coe, 1984), and indicate that the need characteristics are the most important predictors.

Significant changes in the effects of three of the predisposing, enabling, and need characteristics occur during the course of the study. These involve labor-force participation, life in the West (vs. life in the Midwest), and perceived health status. None of these, however, forms a consistent pattern of change that can be observed with all successive comparisons. For example, the only significant change (a modest decline) in the effect of labor-force participation occurs when the coefficient obtained in the mid-1980s is compared with those obtained in the 1970s. Similarly, the only significant change (again a modest decline) in the effect of living in the West occurs when the coefficient obtained in the mid-1970s is compared with those obtained in the early 1970s or the mid-1980s. The only change that occurs in the effect of perceived health is when the coefficient obtained in the early 1970s is compared to any of its counterparts (which are equivalent). Thus, although palpable differences occur for these three variables, they most likely represent fluctuations rather than patterned changes.

Examining the effects of the cohort dummies and the intercepts facilitates an assessment of the net effects of age, period, and cohort on the number of nights spent in the hospital. Few of the cohort dummies produced significant effects. Moreover, in the one case

Table 5.10 Unstandardized Regression Coefficients (and Their Standard Errors) Obtained by Predicting the Number of Nights Spent in the Hospital During Past Year (Among Those With Nights), for All Cohorts Combined, by Survey Year*

Independent variables	Survey years			
	1972-73	1976-77	1980-81	1984-85
PREDISPOSING				
Demographic				
Sex	-.482 (.132)	-.401 (.135)		-.505 (.143)
Widowhood	.507 (.178)	.441 (.185)		
Social structure				
Education				
Black	.509 (.247)	.525 (.257)		
Hispanic				
Labor force	-.831 (.169)	-.811 (.174)	-.729 (.178)	-.388 (.195)
Living alone				
ENABLING				
Family				
Income				
Telephone				
Community				
Northeast	.741 (.168)	.455 (.176)	.533 (.181)	.381 (.192)
South		-.493 (.157)		-.364 (.171)
West	-1.365 (.185)	-.956 (.195)	-1.184 (.199)	-1.430 (.208)
Farm	-.616 (.280)		-.856 (.350)	
Central city	.296 (.133)			.332 (.150)
NEED				
Limited activity	1.481 (.141)	1.421 (.148)	1.540 (.150)	1.674 (.154)
Perceived health	-.933 (.139)	-1.307 (.143)	-1.489 (.146)	-1.402 (.153)
COHORT STRUCTURE				
Cohort 2				
Cohort 3		.525 (.219)	.561 (.232)	
Cohort 4		.627 (.236)		
Cohort 5	.663 (.228)			
Cohort 6	.564 (.249)			
Cohort 7				
Cohort 8	1.101 (.393)			
Cohort 9				
Intercept	8.738 (.348)	9.459 (.392)	8.821 (.429)	8.313 (.460)
R^2	.089	.092	.100	.096
N of Cases	6,218	5,868	5,646	5,297

*Coefficients not significantly different from 0 at the .05 probability level or beyond are omitted for clarity.

(cohort 3) in which a cohort dummy produced two significant effects, they are equivalent. Thus, no evidence exists of any aging effects. Similarly, the cohort dummies are all equivalent when age-strata comparisons are made within columns. Thus, no evidence exists of any cohort effects either.

Some evidence of period effects exists, however. The intercept obtained for the mid-1970s is significantly larger than that obtained from the mid-1980s. Although the coefficient for the intervening period is not significantly different from either of them it does fall in between. This reflects a monotonic decline in the number of nights spent in the hospital, all other things being equal, from the mid-1970s to the mid-1980s (see Havlik et al., 1987). It is not, however, consistent with the anticipated abrupt impact of Medicare's introduction of the PPS system and its associated DRGs (see Wolinsky, 1988). A potential explanation of why the DRG-related drop between the early and mid-1980s is not as dramatic as expected involves measurement issues. The data in Table 5.10 reflect the average, annualized number of days spent in the hospital rather than the average length of stay. As such, it is less sensitive to change.

When taken together, the data in Tables 5.8 through 5.10 clarify the relationship between age and hospital use. No aging effects are found for any of the measures. Similarly, no cohort effects are found for any of the measures. In contrast, period effects are observed in all three tables. With respect to hospital contact, the period effect reflects an increase in the mid-1980s that is entirely consistent with the appearance of DRGs. The period effect for the number of hospital episodes, however, reflects an increase in the 1970s, followed by stable rates throughout the 1980s. Although the period effect for the number of nights spent in the hospital reflects a continuing decline over time, no marked acceleration of that decline is associated with the advent of DRGs, as was expected. Thus, although these data reveal period effects, all of them cannot be readily associated with the implementation of DRGs in the mid-1980s.

AGING, PERIOD, AND COHORT EFFECTS AMONG PREDISPOSING, ENABLING, AND NEED CHARACTERISTICS

Before proceeding to a discussion of the data shown later in Tables 5.11 to 5.19, it would seem appropriate to review briefly how those results were obtained, how they are to be interpreted, and how they were selected for presentation. As indicated at the beginning of this chapter, multivariate regression equations reflecting the behavioral model of the use of health services (again, see Chapter 3 for a detailed review of that model) were separately estimated within each cell of the standard cohort tables. These equations contain all of the measures of the predisposing, enabling, and need characteristics included in Tables 5.1 to 5.10. They do not, however, contain any measures of age. The reason for this is that the equations are estimated separately for each cohort at each point in time. Thus, the equations are cohort and period specific.

The partial, unstandardized regression coefficients (and their standard errors) obtained then become the input data for a new set of cohort tables. This set consists of 156 cohort tables. There is one table for the regression coefficients of each independent variable used to predict each dependent variable. For example, one of these 156 tables contains the partial, unstandardized regression coefficients of income obtained when predicting dental contact rates separately within each cell of the standard cohort table. To simplify matters, the coefficients obtained for those cells belonging to any cohort that enters or leaves the tables after the beginning of the study period are omitted. That is, only complete diagonals are included.

The interpretation of these tables is equivalent to the interpretational methods for traditional cohort analysis (see Chapter 4), with one exception. Instead of the cell entries being the unadjusted means of the dependent variable, the cell entries are the partial, unstandardized regression coefficients of that independent variable on that dependent variable. As such, the interpretation is whether the structural relationship between the two variables is stable, or subject to age, period, or cohort effects. To identify such effects, these tables are visually and statistically inspected by making the appropriate diagonal (i.e., aging), row (i.e., period), and column (i.e., cohort) comparisons. As in traditional cohort analysis, these comparisons are subject to the same confounding effects. That is, the diagonal comparisons reflect both aging and period effects, the row comparisons reflect both period and cohort effects, and the column comparisons reflect both cohort and aging effects.

Although all 156 of these tables were carefully scrutinized, they are not all presented here. Instead, only the 9 tables containing any discernible patterns are presented and discussed. The reason for this is that most of the structural relationships examined are rather stable. Indeed, the 147 tables not presented do no reveal consistent patterns either at the successive comparison (i.e., adjacent cells) level, or at the level of the beginning and end of the comparison string (i.e., diagonal, row, or column). The tables that are presented are discussed in four groups based on commonalities in terms of the independent or dependent variables involved. This is followed by a brief commentary on 6 other tables (not presented) that are somewhat suggestive of possible patterns.

Effect of Income on Dental Contact Rates

Table 5.11 contains the partial, unstandardized regression coefficients of income obtained when predicting dental contact rates. Significant positive effects are obtained for every cell, with two exceptions. Those involve the oldest cohort in the mid-1970s and early 1980s, where the effects are positive but not significantly different from 0. Thus, these results reveal important income barriers to dental contact rates. Regardless of what cohort one selects or which period one considers, individuals with higher family incomes are more likely to have seen a dentist at least once during the past 12 months than their counterparts with lower family incomes.

The important question here, however, is whether the effect of family income on dental contact rates is subject to aging, period, or cohort effects. Answering that question requires the diagonal, row, and column examination of the coefficients in Table 5.11, both in terms of adjacent cell (successive) comparisons, and in terms of the beginning and end of the comparison strings. The diagonal string comparisons yield significant increases in the effects of family income for the five youngest cohorts, with 8 of the 10 successive comparisons involving those cohorts yielding significant differences as well. Moreover, of all the diagonal comparisons in the table, only 3 successive comparisons fail to reflect the consistent monotonic trend of the increasing importance of income on dental contact rates as the cohorts age. Thus, it would appear that a significant pattern of aging effects has been detected, at least for the younger cohorts.

As indicated earlier (see especially Chapter 4), however, the aging effects reflected in diagonal comparisons are confounded by the presence of period effects. Therefore, before much confidence can be placed in the interpretation of the diagonal comparisons as aging effects, the row comparisons must also be made. The row comparisons complicate matters considerably. The row string comparisons indicate significant increases in the effect of income on dental contact for six of the eight age-groups, with 10 of the 11 successive compari-

Table 5.11 Partial, Unstandardized Regression Coefficients (and Standard Errors) Obtained for Family Income From Predicting Dental Contact During Past Year, by Survey Year and Age-Group

Age-group	Survey year		
	1972-73	1976-77	1980-81
56-59	.078 (.005)		
60-63	.070 (.006)	.100 (.008)	
64-67	.077 (.006)	.094 (.009)	.165 (.012)
68-71	.096 (.007)	.118 (.010)	.162 (.013)
72-75	.084 (.009)	.105 (.011)	.148 (.015)
76-79	.082 (.010)	.088 (.013)	.150 (.018)
80-83	.057 (.012)	.096 (.016)	.161 (.022)
84-87	.073 (.016)	.051 (.020)	.109 (.026)
88-91		.059 (.033)	.100 (.045)
92-95			.143 (.077)

sons involving those age-groups significant as well. Moreover, of all of the row comparisons in Table 5.11, only one fails to reflect the monotonic increase in the effect of income. Thus, the row comparisons suggest the presence of considerable period effects. Because considerable overlap exists between the cells involved in the diagonal and row comparisons, determining whether these differences reflect aging or period effects (or both) requires an examination of the column comparisons, inasmuch as the row comparisons are confounded by cohort effects as well.

It is, indeed, the column comparisons that simplify the interpretation of the effects noted in Table 5.11. None of the column string comparisons reveal any significant differences, and only 5 of the 21 successive comparisons within columns yield significant differences. Those successive comparisons, however, do not form a consistent pattern. Thus, no evidence exists of age-strata (cohort) differences.

Because age-strata differences reflect both cohort and aging effects, the absence of age-strata differences indicates that the diagonal differences result from period effects rather than aging effects. The effect of income on dental contact rates simply becomes more important during the study period. This is consistent with the results presented in Table 5.5 with one exception. Those analyses suggested an interaction between age and period that was interpreted such that the oldest-old fared worse than their younger counterparts in terms of the increasing economic barriers associated with double-digit inflation (see Wolinsky & Arnold, 1989). These data, however, indicate that this is not the case, at least with respect to the effect of income. This discontinuity between the two analyses may result more from the measurement limitations in the HISs regarding financial barriers than from anything else.

Effect of Limited Activity on Physician Use

Table 5.12 contains the partial, unstandardized regression coefficients of limited activity owing to health reasons obtained when predicting physician contact rates. With the exception of 5 of the 32 cells, the effect of limited activity is positive and significant. The exceptions all involve the oldest cohorts, which produce positive, but not significant, effects. Thus, these data reveal an important and intuitively pleasing pattern. Individuals who have limited activity because of health reasons are more likely to see a physician at least once a year than are their more fortunate counterparts.

The diagonal string comparisons yield significant differences reflecting a declining effect of limited activity as each of the five youngest cohorts age. Only four of the successive comparisons along the diagonals, however, yield significant differences. Moreover, three of these involve the last column of data, which is precisely when the NCHS introduced the instrumentation changes involving the limited activity question into the HISs. Accordingly, although a gradual decline in the effect of limited activity was detected by the diagonal string comparisons, the bulk of that effect (in terms of significant successive comparisons) appears to be the result of the instrumentation change rather than a meaningful aging effect. Indeed, when the diagonal string comparisons are restricted to the first three columns of

Table 5.12 Partial, Unstandardized Regression Coefficients (and Standard Errors) Obtained for Limited Activity From Predicting Physician Contact During Past Year, by Survey Year and Age-Group

Age-group	Survey year			
	1972-73	1976-77	1980-81	1984-85
56-59	.180 (.013)			
60-63	.159 (.013)	.154 (.013)		
64-67	.159 (.013)	.148 (.013)	.157 (.013)	
68-71	.134 (.013)	.138 (.013)	.133 (.013)	.116 (.013)
72-75	.135 (.014)	.139 (.014)	.127 (.014)	.118 (.014)
76-79	.120 (.016)	.149 (.017)	.123 (.016)	.055 (.016)
80-83	.112 (.021)	.098 (.021)	.084 (.021)	.069 (.019)
84-87	.100 (.030)	.100 (.030)	.178 (.028)	.059 (.026)
88-91		.016 (.055)	.090 (.049)	.081 (.040)
92-95			.139 (.100)	.081 (.104)
96-99				.429 (.264)

data (to eliminate any artifact associated with the instrumentation changes), only two of the five cohorts exhibit significant differences. Thus, there do not appear to be any meaningful aging effects in Table 5.12.

The row comparisons reveal a somewhat similar situation. Significant row string comparisons are found only for the 76 to 79 and 80 to 83 age-groups. Only one significant successive comparison exists, however, and it involves the last column as well. When the row string comparisons are restricted to the first three columns, no significant differences are found. Therefore, the effect of limited activity owing to health reasons on physician contact rates appears to be rather stable across periods.

A similar story is told by the age-strata comparisons within columns. Although the column string comparisons yield significant differences for the early and mid-1970s, only one successive comparison is found. Moreover, 5 of the 16 successive comparisons involved in these two columns break with the expected monotonic pattern of decline. Therefore, for all intents and purposes, the effect of limited activity on physician contact rates appears to be rather stable across cohorts.

Table 5.13 contains the partial, unstandardized regression coefficients of limited activity owing to health reasons obtained from predicting the number of physician visits during the past 12 months, among those with at least one visit. In all but five cells, the effect is significant and positive, indicating that individuals with activity limitations go to the physician more often than their more fortunate counterparts. The exceptions involve the oldest cohorts, whose coefficients are positive but not significant. As was the case with Table 5.12, these results are intuitively pleasing and consistent with those reported earlier in this chapter.

The diagonal string comparisons yield significant differences only for the two youngest cohorts. Moreover, only two of the successive comparisons involving these two cohorts reflect significant differences. Aside from these two cohorts, only three other successive comparisons reveal significant differences. Thus, little or no evidence exists of any consistent pattern of aging effects on the relationship between limited activity and the number of physician visits.

This is not at all consistent with a previously published preliminary report from this study (see Wolinsky et al., 1988). In fact, it is because of this disjuncture that Table 5.13 is presented and discussed here. The prior report found that not only did the effect of limited activity decline as the cohorts aged, but that the decline accelerated among the oldest cohorts. The reason for the disjuncture between the two reports lies in the manner in which limited activity was coded. In the prior report limited activity was coded into four ordered categories reflecting the degree of the activity limitation. In the present analysis limited activity is dichotomized into no activity limitations versus some activity limitations, based on the belief that this more accurately captures the essence of the distinction (see Chapter 2). Although the dichotomous version used here may be the most defen-

Table 5.13 Partial, Unstandardized Regression Coefficients (and Standard Errors) Obtained for Limited Activity From Predicting Number of Physician Visits During Past Year (Among Those With Visits), by Survey Year and Age-Group

Age-group	Survey year			
	1972-73	1976-77	1980-81	1984-85
56-59	2.143 (.120)			
60-63	1.978 (.123)	2.132 (.124)		
64-67	1.888 (.128)	2.110 (.127)	1.736 (.126)	
68-71	1.679 (.139)	1.796 (.136)	1.611 (.133)	1.822 (.138)
72-75	1.600 (.159)	1.860 (.156)	1.592 (.153)	1.583 (.154)
76-79	1.399 (.188)	1.352 (.192)	1.269 (.184)	1.719 (.176)
80-83	1.053 (.238)	1.466 (.229)	1.151 (.233)	1.503 (.229)
84-87	.552 (.352)	.879 (.356)	.830 (.312)	1.326 (.298)
88-91		1.722 (.605)	.569 (.525)	1.547 (.481)
92-95			1.784 (1.200)	1.849 (1.153)
96-99				.142 (3.949)

sible based on logical grounds, the polytomous version used earlier appears to be more sensitive to change.

The row comparisons also fail to yield significant patterns. Only the row string comparison for the 84 to 87 age-group reveals a significant difference. That increase, however, is gradual, and does not result in any significant successive comparisons. Indeed, the only two significant successive comparisons that occur across the rows are separated by two age-groups and involve different periods. Thus, in the absence of any other consistent row effects, no period effects appear to be in Table 5.13.

The age-strata comparisons within columns reveal a similar situation. Only the column string comparison for the early 1970s reveals a significant difference. No significant successive comparisons, however, are in that column. Indeed, the three significant successive comparisons that do occur in Table 5.13 are found in the mid-1970s, although the column string comparison for that period is not significant. Accordingly, the effect of limited activity on the number of physician visits appears to be relatively stable across cohorts.

When taken together, then, the data in Tables 5.12 and 5.13 do not indicate the presence of any aging, period, or cohort effects on the relationship between limited activity and physician use. This holds regardless of whether the measure of physician use involves physician contact or the number of visits (among those with at least one visit). The stability of the relationship between limited activity and physician use calls into question previous reports suggesting that older adults begin to discount their response (in terms of going to see a physician) to activity limitations because those limitations are viewed as a natural part of the aging process (see Ferraro, 1980; Fillenbaum, 1979; Wolinsky et al., 1988). Further research with more precise, reliable, and valid measures of limited activity, however, will be needed to resolve this issue.

Effects of Perceived Health

Tables 5.14, 5.15, and 5.16 contain the partial, unstandardized regression coefficients of perceived health obtained from predicting the taking of restricted activity days, the taking of bed disability days, and hospital contact, respectively. They are simultaneously presented and discussed here because of the similarity in the patterns that they contain. With the exception of 10 of the 96 cells, all of which involve the two oldest cohorts, the effect of perceived health status on these three measures of the use of health services is always negative and significant. Individuals who perceive themselves to be in excellent or good health are significantly less likely to take restricted activity or bed disability days during the past two weeks, or to have been hospitalized during the past 12 months than are their counterparts who perceive themselves to be in fair or poor health. This is both consistent with the findings reported earlier in this chapter, and intuitively pleasing as well.

Table 5.14 Partial, Unstandardized Regression Coefficients (and Standard Errors) Obtained for Perceived Health From Predicting the Taking of Restricted Activity Days During Past 2 Weeks, by Survey Year and Age-Group

Age-group	Survey year			
	1972-73	1976-77	1980-81	1984-85
56-59	-.135 (.009)			
60-63	-.122 (.010)	-.141 (.011)		
64-67	-.116 (.010)	-.142 (.011)	-.147 (.012)	
68-71	-.135 (.011)	-.132 (.012)	-.163 (.013)	-.137 (.011)
72-75	-.156 (.013)	-.158 (.014)	-.170 (.014)	-.151 (.013)
76-79	-.149 (.015)	-.125 (.017)	-.155 (.017)	-.150 (.015)
80-83	-.166 (.019)	-.144 (.021)	-.178 (.022)	-.178 (.021)
84-87	-.191 (.029)	-.157 (.030)	-.191 (.029)	-.169 (.027)
88-91		-.138 (.054)	-.175 (.046)	-.158 (.043)
92-95			.060 (.104)	-.318 (.088)
96-99				.098 (.299)

The diagonal string comparisons reveal an interesting pattern that is remarkably consistent in Tables 5.14 through 5.16. Significant increases in the effect of perceived health are found for cohorts 2 through 4. It is only for the taking of bed disability days, however, that significant successive comparisons are observed for these three cohorts. Even then, this is not the case for all of the successive

Table 5.15 Partial, Unstandardized Regression Coefficients (and Standard Errors) Obtained for Perceived Health From Predicting the Taking of Bed Disability Days During the Past 2 Weeks, by Survey Year and Age-Group

Age-group	Survey year			
	1972-73	1976-77	1980-81	1984-85
56-59	-.068 (.007)			
60-63	-.064 (.007)	-.072 (.008)		
64-67	-.068 (.007)	-.087 (.008)	-.061 (.008)	
68-71	-.064 (.008)	-.081 (.008)	-.067 (.009)	-.081 (.009)
72-75	-.090 (.009)	-.098 (.010)	-.072 (.010)	-.100 (.010)
76-79	-.086 (.011)	-.065 (.012)	-.064 (.012)	-.101 (.012)
80-83	-.115 (.014)	-.110 (.015)	-.117 (.016)	-.135 (.016)
84-87	-.137 (.022)	-.136 (.022)	-.108 (.022)	-.134 (.022)
88-91		-.079 (.042)	-.089 (.032)	-.134 (.035)
92-95			.096 (.079)	-.282 (.086)
96-99				-.064 (.198)

comparisons. Thus, the increasing effect of perceived health appears to be rather gradual and limited to these younger cohorts.

At the same time, however, some suggestive evidence exists for a similar yet weaker aging effect among the other cohorts. That is, with two exceptions, all of the other diagonal string comparisons in Tables 5.14 through 5.16 reflect an increase in the effect of perceived health, although none of those increases is statistically significant. This may indicate that the increasing importance of perceived health associated

with the aging of the cohorts is a more uniform and gradual phenomenon among the elderly that is sharply accelerated when the cohorts
enter and pass through their sixth decade. Such an interpretation
would be consistent with either an anticipatory role socialization
perspective (see Rosow, 1985), or the acceptance of the inevitability
or normative aspects of poor health associated with being elderly (see
Ferraro, 1980; Fillenbaum, 1979). Neither of these interpretations
can be explored further, however, without access to additional col-

Table 5.16 Partial, Unstandardized Regression Coefficients (and Standard Errors) Obtained for Perceived Health From Predicting Hospital Contact During Past Year, by Survey Year and Age-Group

Age-group	Survey year			
	1972-73	1976-77	1980-81	1984-85
56-59	-.095 (.009)			
60-63	-.092 (.010)	-.096 (.010)		
64-67	-.091 (.011)	-.089 (.012)	-.088 (.012)	
68-71	-.078 (.012)	-.086 (.013)	-.110 (.013)	-.121 (.013)
72-75	-.116 (.014)	-.089 (.015)	-.081 (.016)	-.126 (.015)
76-79	-.093 (.017)	-.116 (.018)	-.138 (.018)	-.128 (.018)
80-83	-.131 (.020)	-.105 (.024)	-.112 (.024)	-.147 (.024)
84-87	-.097 (.031)	-.070 (.033)	-.155 (.032)	-.124 (.033)
88-91		-.058 (.057)	-.051 (.049)	-.151 (.050)
92-95			.067 (.104)	-.183 (.122)
96-99				-.418 (.371)

umns of data (beyond the mid-1980s) so that the behavior of these (as well as other) younger cohorts can be observed as they enter and exit their seventh and eighth decades.

That such a pattern of aging effects involves the relationship between perceived health and these three measures of use of health services warrants further comment. The taking of restricted activity or bed disability days, and having been hospitalized all have a common theme. They all involve the recognition of a health problem so significantly troubling that it requires a significant reduction in one's normal role activities (i.e., lost or reduced days of productivity). This commonality provides further support for the two interpretations advanced earlier, inasmuch as they both focused on role changes and the individual's adjustment to those changes. Accordingly, confidence in the preceding interpretations is increased.

The row comparisons in Tables 5.14 through 5.16 fail to reveal any consistent period effects. Indeed, only three of the row string comparisons indicate significant differences, none of these involve the same age-group, and only two occur in the same table. Moreover, of the 63 successive comparisons, only 14 yield significant differences, only 1 of which occurs within the 3 significant string comparisons. Therefore, no palpable (or suggestive) period effects exist in these three tables. This provides further support for the aging effects described earlier, inasmuch as those diagonal comparisons were potentially confounded by period effects.

Similarly, the column comparisons fail to reveal any consistent cohort effects. Only one of the column string comparisons is significant (the early 1970s for the taking of bed disability days). Of the 84 successive comparisons, only 16 indicate significant differences, with no more than 2 occurring in any given column. Therefore, no palpable (or suggestive) cohort effects occur in Tables 5.14 through 5.16 either.

Prediction of Perceived Health

Table 5.17 contains the partial, unstandardized regression coefficients of being a woman obtained when predicting perceived health. Only eight of the cells contain significant effects, all but one of which indicate that women are more likely to perceive their health to be excellent or good than are men. This is at one and the same time both expected and unexpected based on the results reported earlier in this chapter. It is consistent in terms of the direction of the effect. It is inconsistent, however, in terms of the large number of cells that do

Table 5.17 Partial, Unstandardized Regression Coefficients (and Standard Errors) Obtained for Being a Woman From Predicting Perceived Health, by Survey Year and Age-Group

Age-group	Survey year			
	1972-73	1976-77	1980-81	1984-85
56-59	.090 (.010)			
60-63	.085 (.011)	.079 (.011)		
64-67	.017 (.012)	.029 (.012)	.040 (.012)	
68-71	.003 (.013)	.021 (.014)	.037 (.014)	.036 (.014)
72-75	-.026 (.016)	-.014 (.017)	.006 (.016)	.024 (.017)
76-79	.002 (.019)	.002 (.020)	.025 (.021)	-.035 (.021)
80-83	-.015 (.024)	-.049 (.026)	-.045 (.026)	-.030 (.028)
84-87	-.014 (.035)	.040 (.037)	-.030 (.036)	-.030 (.037)
88-91		-.096 (.059)	-.017 (.063)	-.140 (.061)
92-95			-.031 (.114)	.087 (.131)
96-99				.220 (.210)

not reveal an effect. That explains why the age-general coefficients reported in Table 5.1 are much smaller than several of the significant coefficients shown here (owing to the averaging of the insignificant age-specific coefficients into the age-general coefficient).

The diagonal comparisons reveal a rather limited but marked pattern. Significant diagonal string differences are found only for the three youngest cohorts, all of which indicate a decline and virtual elimination of the gender gap in perceived health. Nearly all of that decline, however, is precipitously associated with the successive comparisons involved as the cohorts move into the retirement years (i.e., as they reach their mid-60s). This is consistent with the fixed-role obligation hypothesis (see Marcus & Seeman, 1981a, 1981b; Marcus & Siegel, 1982) and suggests that the perceived health status of men becomes much more like that of women, once the men retire. The interpretation provided by that hypothesis focuses on the reduction in fixed-role obligations brought about retirement, which permits a relatively rapid adjustment of relative self-assessments such as perceived health.

Because the detection of aging effects is potentially confounded by period effects, the preceding interpretation must be considered tentative until the row comparisons have been made. The row string comparisons reveal significant changes only for the 68 to 71 and 72 to 75 age-groups. Both of these changes indicate an increase in the gender gap. Those increases, however, are not palpable at the successive comparison level. Moreover, only two of the eight cells involved contain significant coefficients. Thus, no meaningful period effects are in Table 5.17. This finding provides further confidence for the interpretation of the aging effects presented earlier.

The age-strata comparisons reveal what appear to be cohort effects (that are subject to confounding by aging effects). Significant differences are found for the column string comparisons for the 1970s, but not for the 1980s. The bulk of the changes reflected in these comparisons, however, involves the successive comparisons between the 60 to 63 and 64 to 67 age-groups. These changes reflect aging and not cohort effects because: (a) they are precisely the age-groups involved in the pattern of aging effects described earlier; (b) in the early 1970s no other significant successive comparisons exist; and (c) in the mid-1970s the direction of the changes indicated by the four other significant successive comparisons oscillates. This provides further confidence in the interpretation of the aging effects presented earlier.

Table 5.18 contain partial, unstandardized regression coefficients of living alone obtained from predicting perceived health. Twenty-six of the 32 cells yield significant coefficients, all of which are positive. This is consistent with the results reported earlier in this chapter, as well as with the extant literature (see Cafferata, 1987; Homan, Haddock, Winner, Coe, & Wolinsky, 1986). It reflects the fact that for elderly individuals to live alone they must be in relatively good health.

The diagonal comparisons reveal a rather limited and modest pattern of aging effects. Significant diagonal string comparisons are ob-

Table 5.18 Partial, Unstandardized Regression Coefficients (and Standard Errors) Obtained for Living Alone From Predicting Perceived Health, by Survey Year and Age-Group

Age-group	Survey year			
	1972-73	1976-77	1980-81	1984-85
56-59	-.002 (.016)			
60-63	.032 (.016)	.033 (.017)		
64-67	.061 (.017)	.077 (.018)	.049 (.018)	
68-71	.099 (.018)	.103 (.020)	.113 (.020)	.079 (.020)
72-75	.128 (.021)	.104 (.022)	.089 (.022)	.116 (.022)
76-79	.184 (.023)	.097 (.026)	.112 (.026)	.135 (.027)
80-83	.116 (.029)	.180 (.031)	.205 (.030)	.133 (.034)
84-87	.069 (.040)	.161 (.043)	.101 (.040)	.205 (.044)
88-91		.128 (.067)	.163 (.072)	.219 (.066)
92-95			.157 (.135)	.362 (.124)
96-99				-.377 (.388)

served but only for the three youngest cohorts. Moreover, even for these cohorts, the only significant successive comparisons all occur at the beginning of the strings. Once again, it would appear that such an aging effect is limited to the transitional changes associated with entering the retirement years (see Marcus & Seeman, 1981a, 1981b; Marcus & Siegel, 1982).

An alternative explanation may also appear plausible. The increase in the effect of living alone on the perceived health status of the youngest cohorts may reflect compositional change (see Chapter 1) occurring in those cohorts. This would be consistent with the notion of a survival effect (see Manton & Soldo, 1985), suggesting that individuals in better health are more likely to live to retirement than their less healthy counterparts. Such an interpretation, however, is not consistent with the fact that all but one of the other diagonal string comparisons reveal generally consistent but not significant monotonic increases in the coefficients as well. Moreover, the literature on survival effects does not indicate a precipitous threshold corresponding to the transition to retirement that is reflected in these data. Accordingly, the plausibility of this interpretation is somewhat diminished.

The row comparisons do not reveal any consistent patterns. Only the row string comparison for the 84 to 87 age-group is significant, indicating an increase over time in the effect of living alone on perceived health. In all of the remaining rows only three successive comparisons are significant, two of which indicate a reduction in the effect of living alone. Accordingly, no meaningful period effects are in Table 5.18. This provides further confidence in the identification of the aging effects described earlier.

None of the column string comparisons yield significant differences. Although 11 of the 28 successive comparisons are significant, no consistent patterns are revealed. Indeed, of the 5 of those significant successive comparisons that occur in the early 1970s, 3 indicate an increase, and 2 indicate a decrease in the effect of living alone on perceived health. Thus, no meaningful cohort differences are in Table 5.18 either.

Table 5.19 contains the partial, unstandardized regression coefficients of family income obtained from predicting perceived health. Significant coefficients are found for 20 of the 32 cells. The absence of many significant coefficients among the oldest-old is primarily a reflection of the smaller sample sizes in those cells. All of significant coefficients indicate that individuals with higher incomes are more likely to perceive themselves to be in excellent or good health than are their counterparts with lower incomes. This is consistent with the results reported earlier in this chapter, as well as with the extant literature (see Ferraro, 1980; Fillenbaum, 1979).

The diagonal comparisons reveal what appears to be a reltively strong aging effect, but only for the three youngest cohorts. For these

Table 5.19 Partial, Unstandardized Regression Coefficients (and Standard Errors) Obtained for Family Income From Predicting Perceived Health, by Survey Year and Age-Group

Age-group	Survey year			
	1972-73	1976-77	1980-81	1984-85
56-59	.067 (.005)			
60-63	.065 (.005)	.083 (.007)		
64-67	.053 (.006)	.076 (.008)	.111 (.011)	
68-71	.053 (.007)	.075 (.009)	.100 (.012)	.161 (.016)
72-75	.036 (.009)	.065 (.011)	.084 (.014)	.116 (.019)
76-79	.049 (.010)	.043 (.013)	.023 (.018)	.116 (.022)
80-83	.039 (.013)	.023 (.016)	.058 (.022)	.034 (.029)
84-87	.026 (.018)	.008 (.023)	.017 (.029)	.028 (.039)
88-91		.069 (.033)	.088 (.053)	.053 (.057)
92-95			.121 (.094)	.065 (.109)
96-99				-.129 (.275)

three cohorts all of the row string comparisons are significant. Moreover, five of their nine successive comparisons are significant as well. All of these comparisons indicate the increasing importance of family income on perceived health. The interpretation of this pattern, however, is rather puzzling.

On the one hand, these are the same cohorts for which aging effects were found regarding the relationship between being a woman, living alone, and perceived health status. That much is comforting. More-over, the fixed role obligations hypothesis (see Marcus & Seeman, 1981a, 1981b; Marcus & Siegel, 1982) that was used to explain those relationships appears to have some appeal in this case as well. That is, the declining income levels associated with the transition to retire-ment could plausibly result in the increasing importance of income on self-assessments of health status.

Conversely, it is difficult to understand why such effects would be limited to those just entering the retirement years. It would seem more plausible if those changes in the effects of income were of a more temporary nature, followed either by stabilization at the new level, or by a return to preretirement levels. Instead, the effect of income continues its progressive climb for these three cohorts. More-over, at comparable age-grades, none of the other cohorts exhibit similar increases.

The row comparisons shed some light on this dilemma. Five of the younger age-groups (i.e., those aged 60 to 63 through 76 to 79) have significant row string comparisons reflecting an increase in the effect of income on perceived health over time. All of the successive com-parisons involving the same cells that appear in the three youngest cohorts' diagonal comparisons reveal significant differences. This sug-gests that the age-related changes described earlier are actually the result of period effects consistently affecting all of the age-groups younger than age 80. That is, with the exception of the oldest age-groups, the effect of income on perceived health has become progres-sively more important. Such an interpretation would be consistent with the fact that the oldest-old have significantly less wealth and liquid assets (see Atkins, 1985; Torrey, 1985), and have a more compressed income distribution than their younger counterparts. As a result of their disadvantaged and more homogeneous status, the period effect is less likely to affect them.

As with Tables 5.17 and 5.18, the column comparisons of Table 5.19 reveal little. Only the early 1970s column string comparison yields a significant difference. Moreover, it contains only two signifi-cant successive comparisons. Thus, no meaningful cohort differences exist in Table 5.19 either.

When taken together, then, Tables 5.17 through 5.19 reveal rela-tively little in the way of aging, period, and cohort effects on the relationships between being a woman, living alone, and having a family income with perceived health. A modest decline occurs in the effect of being a woman, but it is observed only among the three youngest cohorts as they age. Similarly, a more pronounced increase occurs in the effect of living alone, but it is also only observed among the three youngest cohorts as they age. Finally, a marked increase occurs in the effect of income over time but only for those cohorts younger than age 80. Although these three patterns may be interpreted in terms of the fixed-role obligations hypothesis (see Marcus & Seeman, 1981a, 1981b; Marcus & Siegel, 1982), further research is needed before confidence in such an explanation can be expressed.

Other Tables Warranting Brief Mention

In addition to the tables already presented (see Tables 5.11 to 5.19), six other tables contained some age, period, or cohort changes in the regression coefficients obtained from predicting the outcome measures. The magnitude and reproducibility of these changes, however, does not warrant presentation of those tables. Accordingly, they are only briefly described here.

The first two of these tables involve the effects of being a woman and being black on the taking of restricted activity days. In both tables the row string comparisons reveal significant changes in the effects over time for four, nonconsecutive age-groups. Few if any of the successive comparisons yield significant differences. Although the age-groups with such significant comparisons are not the same in both tables, they generally involve the young-old and old-old (i.e., those in their late 60s to early 80s). The rather modest positive effects of being a woman or being black dissipate over time, and are no longer statistically significant at the end of the study period. This suggests an increasing homogeneity in the taking of restricted activity days, at least in terms of ascribed status characteristics. Further comment on such limited and marginal period effects, however, is unwarranted.

The last four tables all involve limited activity owing to health reasons, either as a predictor of the taking of restricted activity and bed disability days, or as an outcome of being a woman or being employed. Depending on the particular table examined, aging and period effects are observed. Virtually all of the observed changes involve comparisons of cells in the third and fourth columns that contain individuals 70 years old or older. Inasmuch as this is precisely the point at which the NCHS introduced instrumentation changes in the limited activity measure involving respondents older than age 69, all of these changes appear to be methodological artifacts. Moreover, in each case the changes reflect the effects of the reduced threshold required to classify an individual as having limited activity. Accordingly, further comment on these tables is also unwarranted.

SUMMARY

This chapter has presented the results of the regression-based cohort analyses of all of the measures of health and health behavior. It began by focusing on the more pristine assessment of the aging, period, and cohort effects. This was facilitated by estimating regression equations reflecting the behavioral model of the use of health services separately within each survey year. The results shown in Tables 5.1 to 5.10 revealed a number of interesting patterns in terms of the measures of health status, the use of informal health services, and the use of formal health services.

Among the health-status measures, no aging or period effects were found for perceived health, but evidence of cohort effects existed. The older cohorts viewed themselves as being in better health than did the younger cohorts. This is consistent with the declining adherence to the more traditional and stoic acceptance of life and health held by older generations. In contrast, aging effects were found for limited activity because of health reasons, but no evidence of period or cohort effects existed. As the five older cohorts aged, they experienced more activity limitations. This is consistent with the progressive physiological deterioration associated with the aging process. Taken together, this suggests that the elderly's more subjective assessments of their health status are relatively stable over their life course, but that their more objective assessments are not.

No meaningful aging, period, or cohort effects were found for the two measures of the use of informal health services. That is, the taking of restricted activity and bed disability days was virtually invariant between cohorts as they aged and passed through different periods. This suggests that the use of informal health services is a uniform phenomenon among the elderly, at least in terms of age-related processes.

A rather different situation emerged from the analysis of dental contact rates. Although no aging or period effects were detected, marked cohort differences were found. The older the cohort, the lower the dental contact rate. This indicates that the age-related changes associated with the use of dentists' services resulted from cohort succession. Younger cohorts having higher dental contact rates were replacing older cohorts having lower dental contact rates. This is consistent with the view that oral health behavior is a relatively stable trait among adults.

The analysis of the measures of physician use significantly clarified the long-standing relationship between age and going to see a physician among older adults. No aging effects were detected for either measure. In contrast, period effects were detected for both. A significant increase occurred in physician contact rates over time, coupled with a significant decrease in the number of physician visits, among those with visits to a physician. These period effects reflect the general increase in access to medical care coupled with the increasing efforts at cost-containment that both occurred during the course of the study. Some modest cohort effects were also found on the volume of physician use. Consistent with their more traditional and stoic values, older cohorts had somewhat fewer visits to physicians.

Similarly, the analysis of the hospital use measures significantly clarified the long-standing relationship between age and going to the hospital. No aging or cohort effects were found for any of the measures, but period effects were detected for each. The period effect for hospital contact indicated an increase in the mid-1980s consistent with the appearance of the PPS and its associated DRGs. In contrast, the period effect for the number of hospital episodes involved an increase in the 1970s, followed by stable rates throughout the 1980s. The period effect for the number of nights spent in the hospital indicated a continued decline over time, with no marked acceleration of that decline associated with the onset of DRGs, as was expected. Thus, although period effects were found for all of the meausres of hospital use, they could not all be readily associated with the implementation of DRGs in the mid-1980s.

In the second section of the chapter attention turned to the assessment of aging, period, and cohort effects on the predisposing, enabling, and need characteristics themselves. This involved estimating the behavioral model separately for each cohort within each survey year. The resulting coefficients were then placed into standard cohort table formats, and these new tables were visually and statistically examined. The analyses of Tables 5.11 to 5.19 revealed six major points.

The first and most important point was the remarkable stability in the effects of the predisposing, enabling, and need characteristics across cohorts as they aged through different periods. Indeed, of the 156 structural relationships examined, only 9 showed any evidence of aging, period, or cohort effects. Several of those relationships were methodological artifacts of the instrumentation changes introduced into the HISs by the NCHS in the mid-1980s involving the questions assessing limited activity owing to health reasons. Accordingly, at the general level, the effects of the predisposing, enabling, and need characteristics were found to be relatively unaffected by aging, period, and cohort phenomena.

Nonetheless, five rather specific effects were detected. The first of these involved the effect of family income on dental contact rates. For all but the oldest age-groups, period effects were found that significantly increased the economic barriers to dental care over time. This confirms the earlier regression-based cohort analysis that identified increasing financial inequities in the oral health care of elderly Americans.

The second effect involved the relationship between perceived health and the taking of restricted activity days, the taking of bed disability days, and having been hospitalized in the past year. In all three cases a significant increase in the effect of perceived health was found as the three youngest cohorts aged. In addition, similar but weaker (and nonsignificant) aging effects were observed for the older cohorts. These effects indicate that the increasing importance of perceived health associated with the aging of the cohorts is a more uniform and gradual phenomenon among the elderly that is sharply accelerated when the cohorts enter and pass through their sixth decade. This is consistent with hypotheses about both the anticipatory role socialization associated with entering the retirement years, and with the acceptance of the inevitability or normative aspects of poor health associated with being elderly.

A third effect involved the relationship between status as a woman and perceived health. In the three preretirement cohorts, an aging effect was detected that resulted in the reduction, if not elimination, of the gender gap. This was interpreted as consistent with the fixed-role obligations hypothesis. It suggests that the perceived health status of men becomes much more like that of women, once the men retire. Presumably, the reduction in fixed-role obligations associated with retirement translates into a rapid adjustment of relative self-assessments, like perceived health.

The fourth effect involved an increase in the importance of living alone on perceived health as the three youngest cohorts aged. That is, as the preretirement cohorts entered the retirement years, the positive relationship between living alone and perceived health became stronger. This, too, was found to be consistent with the fixed-role obligations hypothesis. It suggests that the loss of work-related contacts makes it more difficult for individuals in poorer health to remain sufficiently independent to live alone.

Finally, the fifth effect involves the relationship between family income and perceived health. Here, a period effect was found for the five younger age-groups (i.e., those younger than age 80). Over time, income became more important in terms of perceived health for these age-groups. That it did not increase for the older age-groups is consistent with the fact that the oldest-old have significantly less wealth and liquid assets, and a more compressed income distribution than their younger counterparts. As a result of their disadvantaged status, the period effect did not affect the oldest age-groups.

REFERENCES

Aday, L. A., & Eichhorn, R. (1972). *The utilization of health services: Indices and correlates* (DHEW Publication No. HSM-73-3003). Washington, DC: Government Printing Office.

Aday, L. A., Fleming, G. V., & Andersen, R. M. (1984). *Access to medical care in the U.S.: Who has it, who doesn't.* Chicago: Pluribus Press.

Andersen, R. M. (1968). *A behavioral model of families' use of health services.* Chicago: Center for Health Administration Studies.

Andersen, R. M., Mullner, R. M., & Cornelius, L. J. (1987). Black-white differences in health status: Methods or substance. *Milbank Quarterly, 65* S72–S99.

Andersen, R. M., & Newman, J. (1973). Societal and individual determinants of medical care utilization in the United States. *Milbank Memorial Fund Quarterly, 51*, 95–124.

Atkins, G. L. (1985). The economic status of the oldest old. *Milbank Memorial Fund Quarterly, 63*, 395–419.

Berki, S. E., Wyszewianski, L., Lichtenstein, R., Gimotty, P. Bowlyow, J., Papke, E., Smith, T., Crane, S., & Bromberg, J. (1985). Health insurance coverage of the unemployed. *Medical Care, 23*, 847–854.

Cafferata, G. L. (1987). Marital status, living arrangements, and the use of health services by elderly Americans. *Journal of Gerontology, 43*, 613–619.

Chen, Y. P. (1988). Better options for work and retirement: Suggestions for improving economic security mechanisms for old age. *Annual Review of Gerontology and Geriatrics, 8*, 189–216.

Cornoni-Huntley, J. C., Foley, D. J., White, L. R., Suzman, R., Berkman, L. F., Evans, D. A., & Wallace R. B., (1985). Epidemiology of disability in the oldest old: Methodologic issues and preliminary findings. *Milbank Memorial Fund Quarterly, 63*, 350–376.

Department of Health and Human Services. (1981). *Summary report of the Graduate Medical Education National Advisory Committee* (DHHS Publication No. 81-151). Washington, DC: Government Printing Office.

Elder, G. H. (1974). *Children of the Great Depression.* Chicago: University of Chicago Press.

Elder, G. H. (1975). Age differentiation and the life course. *Annual Review of Sociology, 1*, 165–190.

Elder, G. H., & Liker, J. K. (1982). Hard times in womens' lives: Historical influences across 40 years. *American Journal of Sociology, 88*, 241–269.

Ferraro, K. R. (1980). Self-ratings of health among the old and the old-old. *Journal of Health and Social Behavior, 21*, 377–382.

Fetter, R. B., Shin, J. L., Freeman, J. L., Averill, R. F., & Thompson, J. D. (1980). Case mix definition of diagnosis-related groups. Medical Care, 18, S1–S53.

Fillenbaum, G. G. (1979). Social context and self-assessments of health among the elderly. Journal of Health and Social Behavior, 20, 45–51.

Fries, J. F. (1980). Aging, natural death, and the compression of morbidity. New England Journal of Medicine, 303, 130–135.

Haug, M., & Lavin, B. (1978). Method of payment for medical care and public attitudes toward physician authority. Journal of Health and Social Behavior, 19, 279–291.

Haug, M., & Lavin, B. (1981). Practitioner or patient: Who's in charge? Journal of Health and Social Behavior, 22, 212–229.

Haug, M., & Lavin, B. (1983). Consumerism in medicine: Challenging physician authority. Beverly Hills: Sage Publications.

Havlik, R. J., Liu, B. M., Kovar, M. G., Suzman, R., Feldman, J. J., Harris, T., & Van Nostrand, J. (1987). Health statistics on older persons, 1986 (DHHS Publication No. 87-1409). Washington, DC: Government Printing Office.

Homan, S. M., Haddock, C. C., Winner, C. A., Coe, R. M., & Wolinsky, F. D. (1986). Widowhood, sex, laborforce participation, and the use of physician services by elderly adults. Journal of Gerontology, 41, 793–796.

Illich, I. (1976). Medical nemesis: The expropriation of our health. New York: Pantheon.

Kegeles, S. S. (1963). Why people seek dental care: A test of a conceptual framework. Journal of Health and Health Behavior, 4, 166–175.

Kiyak, A. (1987). An explanatory model of older persons' use of dental services: Implications for health policy. Medical Care, 25, 936–951.

Krause, N. (1988). Gender and ethnicity differences in psychological well-being. Annual Review of Gerontology and Geriatrics, 8, 156–188.

Longino, C. F., & Soldo, B. J., (1987). The graying of America: Implications of life extension for quality of life. In R. Ward & S. Tobin (Eds.), Health in aging: Sociological issues and policy directions (pp. 58-85). New York: Springer.

Manton, K. G., Patrick, C. H., & Johnson, K. W. (1987). Health differentials between blacks and whites: Recent trends in morbidity and mortality. Milbank Quarterly, 65, S129–S199.

Manton, K. G., & Soldo, B. J. (1985). Dynamics of health changes in the oldest old: New perspectives and evidence. Milbank Memorial Fund Quarterly, 63, 206–285.

Marcus, A., & Seeman, T. (1981a). Sex differences in health status: A re-examination of the nurturant role hypothesis. American Sociological Review, 46, 119–123.

Marcus, A., & Seeman, T. (1981b). Sex differences in reports of illness and disability: A preliminary test of the "fixed role obligations" hypothesis. Journal of Health and Social Behavior, 22, 174–182.

Marcus, A., & Siegel, J. (1982). Sex differences in the use of physician services: A preliminary test of the fixed role hypothesis. Journal of Health and Social Behavior, 23, 186–197.

Mechanic, D. (1985). Cost containment and the quality of medical care: Rationing strategies in an era of constrained resources. Milbank Memorial Fund Quarterly, 63, 453–475.

Robinson, P. K., Coberly, S., & Paul. C. E. (1985). Work and retirement. In R. H. Binstock & E. Shanas (Eds.), Handbook of aging and the social sciences (2nd ed.) (pp. 503-527). New York: Van Nostrand Reinhold.

Roscow, I. (1985). Status and role change through the life cycle. In R. H. Binstock & E. Shanas (Eds.), *Handbook of aging and the social sciences* (2nd ed.) (pp. 62-93). New York: Van Nostrand Reinhold.

Shapiro, E., & Tate, R. B. (1989). Is health care use changing? A comparison between physician, hospital, and nursing home and home care use of two elderly cohorts. *Medical Care, 27,* 1002–1014.

Torrey, B. B. (1985). Sharing increasing costs on declining income: The visible dilemma of the invisible aged. *Milbank Memorial Fund Quarterly, 63,* 377–395.

Verbrugge, L. M. (1985). Gender and health: An update on hypotheses and evidence. *Journal of Health and Social Behavior, 26,* 156–182.

Wolinsky, F. D. (1988). *The sociology of health: Principles, practitioners, and issues* (2nd ed.). Belmont, CA: Wadsworth.

Wolinsky, F. D., & Arnold, C. L. (1988). A different perspective on health and health services utilization. *Annual Review of Gerontology and Geriatrics, 8,* 71–101.

Wolinsky, F. D., & Arnold, C. L. (1989). A birth cohort analysis of dental contact among elderly Americans. *American Journal of Public Health, 79,* 47–51.

Wolinsky, F. D., Arnold C. L., & Nallapati, I. V. (1988). Explaining the declining rate of physician utilization among the oldest-old. *Medical Care, 26,* 544–553.

Wolinsky, F. D., & Coe, R. M. (1984). Physician and hospital utilization among elderly adults: An analysis of the health interview survey. *Journal of Gerontology, 39,* 334–341.

Wolinsky, F. D., Coe, R. M., Miller, D. K., Prendergast, J. M., Creel, M. J., & Chavez, M. N. (1983). Health services utilization among the noninstitutionalized elderly. *Journal of Health and Social Behavior, 24,* 325–337.

Wolinsky, F. D., Mosely, R. R., & Coe, R. M. (1986). A cohort analysis of the use of health services by elderly Americans. *Journal of Health and Social Behavior, 27,* 209–219.

Wolinsky, F. D., & Wolinsky, S. R. (1981). Expecting sick role legitimation and getting it. *Journal of Health and Social Behavior, 22,* 229–242.

Chapter 6

Conclusions and Policy Implications

The purpose of this chapter is to summarize the results of the traditional and regression-based cohort analyses, discuss their implications, and in light of them, propose a restructuring of the American health care delivery system. To achieve these goals, the chapter is divided into three major sections. The first focuses on summarizing the results. Special attention is given to reconciling the differences obtained from the traditional and regression-based cohort analyses, as well as to the limitations involved in any analysis of the HIS data.

The implications of these results are the focus of the second section. Five critical issues are addressed including the observance of negligible aging effects, modest period effects, the substantial cohort effects on dental contact rates, increasing income barriers to dental care, and the maximal effect of need as a discriminating factor. The last section focuses on a proposal for restructuring the health care delivery system in light of these findings and their implications. This proposal is based on five precepts including a shift from age-based to need-based criteria, expanded service coverage, the encouragement of prevention as well as health promotion and maintenance, the introduction of a universal and mandatory national health insurance program for all age-groups, and the reliance on primary care physicians as the cornerstones and gatekeepers of the new system.

SUMMARY

Summarizing a complex study such as this, without overwhelming the reader, can be a difficult task. To minimize that risk, the results obtained from the traditional and regression-based cohort analyses are first considered separately. Then, the differences between them are reconciled, before turning to the effects of age, period, and cohort on the structural relationships themselves. This section concludes with a review of the appropriate caveats based on the limitations of the data.

Results of Traditional Cohort Analysis

Table 6.1 contains a summary of the aging, period, and cohort effects obtained from the traditional cohort analysis of all of the measures of health and health behavior reported in Chapter 4. As such, Table 6.1 reflects the results of diagonal, row, and column comparisons of the means of the cells in the standard cohort tables that are *not* adjusted for the predisposing, enabling, and need characteristics. Therefore, any aging, period, or cohort effects shown here are analogous to zero-order effects.

Two general comments warrant brief mention here before conducting a variable-by-variable review of the results summarized in Table 6.1. First, although aging and period effects are detected for most of the variables under study, these effects are generally modest. Indeed, consistently substantial changes are not found for any measure. Second, only one cohort effect was detected, reflecting an uninterrupted and noteworthy increase in dental contact rates associated with cohort succession. When taken together, these two factors suggest that age-related changes in the health and health behavior of elderly Americans is not at all marked. Rather, it is the absence of such age-related changes that is striking.

Among the health-status measures, both aging and period effects were detected. Cohort effects, however, were not. As the cohorts aged, their health status deteriorated. This was marked by declines in perceived health (before stabilization at about age 90) and concomitant increases in limited activity because of health reasons. Over time there was a slow increase in perceived health status among the pre-retirement age-groups, relatively stable perceptions among the young-old, and a slow downward drift among older elderly. Period effects also included a slow increase in limited activity over time for those age-groups younger than age 70.

Table 6.1 Summary of Aging, Period, and Cohort Effects Revealed From Traditional Cohort Analysis

Dependent variable	Aging effect	Period effect	Cohort effect
<u>Health status</u>			
Perceived health	Uninterrupted decline that stabilizes at about age 90	Slow increase for pre-retirement age-groups, stability among younger elderly and a slow downward drift for older elderly	None
Limited activity	Uninterrupted increase for all age-groups	Slow increase for age-groups under 70	None
<u>Informal health services utilization</u>			
Restricted activity days	None	Substantial declines occur for age-groups under 90 between the early and mid 1980s	None
Bed disability days	Slow increase among the young-old	None	None
<u>Dentists' use</u>			
Dental contact	None	None	Uninterrupted increase with cohort succession

Physicians' use		
Physician contact	Slow increase that stabilizes at about age 80	Increase that is strongest for age-groups under 80	None
Physician visits	Slow increase that stabilizes at about age 80, and then begins to decline by about age 90	Consistent decline	None
Hospitals' use		
Hospital contact	Increase that decelerates among the oldest-old	Slow increase among all age-groups	None
Hospital episodes	None	Slow increase among all but the oldest-old	None
Hospital nights	None	Slow decline prior to the mid 1980s among all but the oldest-old, followed by a more dramatic decline during the mid 1980s	None

The results obtained for the measures of informal health services use were even less robust. Neither aging nor cohort effects were found for the taking of restricted activity days. Moreover, although a period effect was observed, reflecting substantial declines in the number of restricted activity days taken by those age-groups younger than age 90, that decline occurred only between the early and mid-1980s. Similarly, neither period nor cohort effects were found for the taking of bed disability days. Although a slow increase was detected as the cohorts aged, that change in the taking of bed disability days was limited to the young-old.

In contrast, the results obtained for dental contact rates were substantial. Although neither aging nor period effects were detected, a rather salient cohort effect was observed. An uninterrupted increase in dental contact rates was clearly associated with cohort succession, such that younger cohorts with higher rates of contact were replacing older cohorts with lower rates of contact. This resulted in a 22% increase in the grand mean of dental contact for these age-groups (i.e., those aged 56 to 99) between the early 1970s and the early 1980s.

The results for physician use revealed a more complex pattern. Aging effects were found for both the contact and number of visits measures. The observed pattern was a slow increase in physician use that stabilized at about age 80. For the physician visits measure, however, a decline in the volume of visits began to occur by about age 90. Period effects were also found for both measures, although the nature of the effects differed. Over time, physician contact rates increased, especially among those age-groups under age 80. During the same period, a consistent decline occurred in the number of physician visits for all age-groups. No cohort effects were found for either measure of physician use.

A similarly complex pattern of effects was found for the measures of hospital use. Aging effects were detected only for hospital contact. These reflected an increase in the likelihood of being hospitalized that decelerated among the oldest-old. In contrast, period effects were detected for all three measures. For hospital contact a slow increase occurred among all age-groups. A comparable increase in the number of hospital episodes was found for all age-groups, except the oldest-old. For the number of nights spent in the hospital, a slow decline was observed before the mid-1980s among all but the oldest-old, followed by a more dramatic decline during the mid-1980s. No cohort effects were detected for any measure of hospital use.

Results of Regression-Based Cohort Analysis

Table 6.2 contains a summary of the aging, period, and cohort effects obtained from the regression-based cohort analysis of all of the measures of health and health behavior reported in Chapter 5. As such, this table reflects the results of the row and column comparisons of the cohort coefficients, as well as the row comparisons of the intercepts. These coefficients were obtained from using the behavioral model (see Andersen, 1968) to predict health and health behavior separately within survey years. Therefore, any aging, period, or cohort effects shown here are analogous to *net* effects, from which the joint effects of the predisposing, enabling, and need characteristics have been separated.

Four general comments warrant brief mention here before proceeding to a variable-by-variable review of the results summarized in Table 6.2. First, the only aging effect that is detected involves limited activity. Second, with the exception of the taking of bed disability days and dental contact rates, period effects are found for every measure of health and health behavior. Third, cohort effects are observed for four variables including perceived health, the taking of restricted activity days, dental contact rates, and the number of physician visits. Finally, unlike the results obtained from the traditional cohort analysis, the regression-based cohort analysis did identify several effects of substantial magnitude.

A relatively complex pattern of aging, period, and cohort effects was found among the health status measures. For perceived health, no aging effects were found. Period and cohort effects, however, were observed. The period effect is such that declines in perceived health occur between the early to mid-1970s and the early to mid-1980s. The cohort effect reflects an uninterrupted decline in perceived health associated with cohort succession that disappears in the mid-1980s. In contrast, aging and period effects were detected for limited activity owing to health reasons, but no cohort effects were found. The aging effect reflects an uninterrupted increase in limited activity for the five older cohorts, whereas the period effect reflects an increase in limited activity for all age-groups.

Little change appears to be occurring among the measures of the use of informal health services. No aging effects are found for either measure. Moreover, although period and cohort effects are found for the taking of restricted activity days, they are not observed for the taking of bed disability days. The period effect reflects a slow decline

Table 6.2 Summary of Aging, Period, and Cohort Effects Revealed From Regression-Based Cohort Analysis

Dependent variable	Aging effect	Period effect	Cohort effect
Health status			
Perceived health	None	Declines between the early to mid 1970s and the early to mid 1980s'	Uninterrupted decline with cohort succession that disappears in the mid 1980s
Limited activity	Uninterrupted increase for the five older cohorts	Increase for all age-groups	None
Use of informal health services			
Restricted activity days	None	Very slow decline	Increase with cohort succession
Bed disability days	None	None	None
Dentists' utilization			
Dental contact	None	None	Uninterrupted increase with cohort succession

Physicians' use

Physician contact	None	Consistent increase	None
Physician visits	None	Consistent decline	Modest increase with cohort succession

Hospitals' use

Hospital contact	None	Substantial increase occurs between the early and mid 1980s	None
Hospital episodes	None	Increase occurred in the early 1970s, followed by rather stable rates thereafter	None
Hospital nights	None	Decline from the mid 1970s to to mid 1980s	None

over time in the number of restricted activity days taken, whereas the cohort effect reflects a modest increase in the taking of restricted activity days associated with cohort succession.

As was the case in the traditional cohort analysis, neither aging nor period effects were detected for dental contact rates. A substantial cohort effect, however, was observed. It reflects an uninterrupted increase in dental contact rates associated with cohort succession. Older cohorts having lower levels of dental contact are being replaced by younger cohorts having higher levels of dental contact. Differences in the magnitude of the cohort coefficients range between 3- and 10-fold when contrasting the youngest and oldest cohorts.

The results obtained for the measures of physician use are, at one and the same time, both easy and difficult to summarize. On the easy side, no aging effects are found for either measure. On the more difficult side, a period effect reflecting a consistent increase in physician contact rates is observed for all age-groups, whereas a period effect reflecting a consistent decline in the number of physician visits is observed for all age-groups. Similarly, although no cohort effect is found for physician contact, an effect reflecting a modest increase associated with cohort succession occurs for the number of physician visits.

A more pristine pattern of effects emerges for the measures of hospital use. Neither aging nor cohort effects are observed for hospital contact, the number of hospital episodes, or the number of nights spent in the hospital. In contrast, period effects are detected for all three measures. The period effect on hospital contact rates shows that a substantial increase occurs between the early and mid-1980s. Similarly, the period effect on the number of hospital episodes also reflects an increase during the early 1970s. That increase, however, is followed by rather stable rates thereafter. In contrast, the period effect on the number of nights spent in the hospital reflects a decline from the mid-1970s to the mid-1980s. Thus, although hospital contact and episode rates rise over the course of the study, average, annually aggregated lengths of stay decline.

Reconciliation of Differences From Traditional and Regression-Based Cohort Analytic Techniques

Even a casual comparison of the results summarized in Tables 6.1 and 6.2 indicates significant differences between the two. On the one hand, the traditional cohort analysis found rather widespread aging and period effects of modest magnitude, coupled with the absence of cohort effects (except for dental contact rates). Conversely, the regression-based cohort analysis found rather widespread period effects and a number of cohort effects, several of which were substantial, coupled with the absence of aging effects (except for limited activity owing to health reasons).

An accounting for these discrepancies lies in the fundamental difference between the two techniques. The traditional cohort analysis reported in Chapter 4 compares and contrasts the means on the dependent variable under scrutiny for each cell in the standard cohort table. For example, the cell entries in Table 4.6 are the means for physician contact for those particular age-groups in those particular survey years. The cell means are not adjusted (or standardized) for any of the predisposing, enabling, or need characteristics contained in the behavioral model (see Andersen, 1968). Thus, any aging, period, or cohort effects identified in the traditional cohort analysis represent zero-order effects.

In contrast, the regression-based cohort analysis reported in Chapter 5 effectively compares and contrasts the means on the dependent variable under scrutiny after adjusting (via multiple regression partialing techniques) for all of the predisposing, enabling, and need characteristics in the behavioral model. For example, differences obtained by comparing and contrasting the cohort coefficients and the intercepts in Table 5.6 represent the adjusted effects of age, period, and cohort on physician contact rates. Accordingly, the regression-based cohort analysis identifies the *net* aging, period, and cohort effects that are not shared (or joint) with the other factors known to affect health and health behavior. As such, any aging, period, or cohort effects identified in the regression-based cohort analysis represent unique effects.

In situations in which the other factors tht affect the health and health behavior of elderly Americans are correlated with age, there will be differences between the zero-order and unique effects of age, period, and cohort. The magnitude of those differences will vary directly with the degree of correlation between age and the other factors. Continuing with the example of physician contact rates, note that the difference observed between the traditional and regression-based cohort analyses involves the presence or absence of aging effects. When the predisposing, enabling, and need factors are not considered, an aging effect is observed. When these other factors are included in the regression analysis, however, no aging effect is found.

The bulk of this difference occurs because physician contact rates are sensitive to health status, which is highly correlated with age. Therefore, if the cell means are not adjusted for health status, then the standard cohort table yields an aging effect, because the joint effects of health status are improperly credited to age. But, when health status and the other factors are considered, only the unique effect of aging is credited to age, which in this case is zero (or no effect).

Similar situations occur regarding the detection (or absence of) aging effects for the taking of bed disability days, the number of physician visits, and hospital contact rates. The traditional cohort analysis identifies aging effects on all three of these variables, whereas the regression-based cohort analysis fails to identify any aging effects on them. Here, again, it is the adjustment for health status that accounts for the bulk of the difference. As indicated earlier, health status is correlated with age. In the absence of adjustments for health status, age appears to be correlated with these measures of health services use. The spuriousness of that association, however, becomes apparent when measures of health status are introduced into the equation.

Among the measures of informal and formal health services use, only two other differences occur between the results of the traditional and regression-based cohort analyses. These involve the absence of cohort effects for the taking of restricted activity days and the number of physician visits when the zero-order effects are estimated versus the presence of cohort effects for these variables when the unique effects are estimated. It is important to note that in both cases the differences are small, with only modest increases associated with cohort succession being detected. Nonetheless, differences are observed.

Accounting for these differences involves the same general logic used to understand those associated with the relationship between age and health status. Here, however, the relationships involve the cohorts and their distributions on the predisposing and enabling characteristics, as well as on the need characteristics. Rather than the cohort effects being the spurious result of the joint relationships involved, they are actually suppressed in the absence of the predisposing, enabling, and need characteristics. That is, an underlying dimension (or more) differentiates the cohorts from each other in terms of their taking of restricted activity days and the number of physician visits.

That dimension, however, is not well tapped (i.e., represented) by any of the predisposing, enabling, or need characteristics. Nonetheless, in the absence of those characteristics from the adjustment process, the underlying dimension that differentiates the cohorts is not palpable. It is only after the adjustment process occurs that the cohort dummies are able to tap the differentiating dimension success-fully. This suggests that the differentiating dimension involves some-thing unique in the life experiences of the cohorts that is substantially unrelated to the characteristics included in the adjustment process. This points to social psychological rather than biological factors, consistent with the relatively stable cohort traits associated with the children of the Great Depression and World War II (see Elder, 1974, 1975; Elder & Liker, 1982).

Further support for this reconciliation of the differences obtained from the traditional and regression-based cohort analyses can be found by focusing on the results obtained for dental contact rates. On the one hand, neither technique detects either aging or period effects. Conversely, both techniques identify cohort effects that reflect an uninterrupted increase in dental contact rates associated with cohort succession. The agreement in the results obtained from the different techniques is understandable when two factors are considered. First, there has never been any clear-cut evidence of aging or period effects on dental contact rates (see Wolinsky & Arnold, 1989). Second, because the known correlates of dental contact rates (i.e., gender, education, income, and living arrangements) have so little impact (see Kiyak, 1987), they do not suppress the underlying dimension that differentiates the cohorts' oral health behavior. As a result, both the traditional and regression-based cohort analytic techniques identify the same cohort succession effect, in the absence of either aging or period effects.

Additional support for the reconciliation of the observed differ-ences obtained from the two techniques can be found by examining the results for the health status measures. On the one hand, no differences are found for limited activity owing to health reasons. This is understandable inasmuch as limited activity taps more objective assessments of health status that are well known to be correlated with age and period (see Cornoni-Huntley et al., 1985). Moreover, these age-related associations are also known not to be significantly reduced by adjustments for the predisposing and enabling characteristics (see Manton & Soldo, 1985). Therefore, it is not surprising that compara-ble aging, period, and cohort effects (or non effects) on limited activity are obtained from the two techniques.

Conversely, significant differences are obtained when the two tech-niques are applied to the perceived health-status measure. The tradi-tional cohort analysis yields an aging effect and a curvilinear period effect, both in the absence of any cohort effect. In contrast, the regression-based cohort analysis yields no aging effect, coupled with consistent period and cohort effects. The difference regarding the aging effect once again involves a spurious zero-order relationship. Several of the predisposing and enabling characteristics including sex, education, living arrangements, and income are related to age. At the same time, these factors are also known correlates of perceived health status (see Ferraro, 1980; Fillenbaum, 1979). Once they are considered, no unique aging effect exists.

Similarly, the difference between the curvilinear period effect on perceived health status identified in the traditional cohort analysis and the consistent period effect identified in the regression-based cohort analysis results from the adjustment process. The dissimilar slope of the curvilinear relationship among the younger elderly disappears when adjustments are made for sex, education, income, and living arrangements. The reason is that younger-elderly have favored status on these factors. When this is considered, a more consistent period effect is estimated.

The difference in the estimation (or lack thereof) of the cohort effect for perceived health status across the two techniques is comparable with that described earlier for the taking of restricted activity days and the number of physician visits. That is, an underlying dimension differentiates the cohorts from each other in terms of their perceived health status. That dimension, however, is not well tapped by any of the predisposing and enabling characteristics. Nonetheless, in the absence of controlling for those characteristics, the underlying dimension that differentiates the perceived health status of the cohorts is not palpable. Again, this suggests that the differentiating dimension most likely consists of social psychological factors consistent with the relatively stable traits associated with the children of the Great Depression and World War II (see Elder, 1974, 1975; Elder & Liker, 1982).

Ultimately, this reconciliation of the two cohort techniques is of considerable importance for two reasons. The first is that it demonstrates the differential utility of the two techniques. In particular, it underscores the advantages of the more pristine assessments of aging, period, and cohort effects obtained from the regression-based cohort analysis. As indicated earlier, this is especially important when other factors, like health status, are jointly correlated with both age and the use of health services. Under such circumstances, traditional cohort analysis, which only yields zero-order effects, produces misleading estimates of the effects of aging. Also as indicated earlier, traditional cohort analysis yields misleading estimates of cohort effects in situa-

tions in which the variables used in the adjustment process suppress
the identification of an underlying dimension that differentiates the
cohorts.

When taken together, these limitations indicate that traditional cohort analysis is not a robust technique for use in situations in which
other important factors having either joint or suppressive relationships
with age and cohort exist. Inasmuch as situations like this are rather
likely to occur in studying the health and health behavior of elderly
Americans, the regression-based cohort technique has a considerable
advantage for the pristine estimation of aging, period, and cohort effects. This is not to suggest, however, that traditional cohort analysis
methods should be abandoned altogether. Rather, the analyses reported
here indicate that the traditional cohort methods should be the first
stage of the analysis, followed by the more rigorous regression-based
techniques. Then, careful reconciliation of any differences in the patterns of the effects observed should occur. Used in tandem, the two
techniques provide a considerably more robust analytic program. Moreover, the reconciliation of the two techniques would serve as a further
mechanism for minimizing the acceptance of any relationships that were
merely statistical artifacts, thus enhancing the study's internal validity
(see Glenn, 1976, 1977, 1989; Palmore, 1978).

The second reason that the reconciliation of the differential results
obtained by the two cohort analytic techniques is so important is that
it also enhances the external validity of the study. That is, the reconciliation makes the synthetic (i.e., cross-sequential) longitudinal analysis of the HISs (see Department of Health and Human Services,
1975, 1985) consistent with the panel analysis of the Manitoba
Longitudinal Study on Aging (MLSA) (see Mossey, Havens, Roos, &
Roos, 1981; Mossey & Shapiro, 1985; Roos & Shapiro, 1981).
Recently, Shapiro and Tate (1989) used log-linear and survival analysis techniques to compare the physician, hospital, nursing home, and
home care services use of two elderly cohorts followed for 8.5 years in
the MLSA. Unlike the earlier report from this study that relied solely
on traditional cohort analysis (see Wolinsky, Mosely, & Coe, 1986),
Shapiro and Tate (1989) found that:

> Aging had little effect on the average number of [physician] visits
> and the very elderly used about the same amount of ambulatory care
> as younger elderly. In fact, in five-year age categories, there was no
> apparent trend from age 65–69 through to 85+. (p. 1011)

Shapiro and Tate (1989) proceed to suggest that the differences
between the two studies stem from the fact that the physician visit

counts in the HIS data were averaged during a 1-year period, whereas
in the MLSA, the physician-visit counts were averaged during an 8.5-
year period. They argue that their "smoothing out" of the annual
variations provides "a more realistic picture" of physician use associated with the aging process.

In contrast, the reconciliation of the two cohort analytic techniques
suggests that the traditional cohort analysis of the HISs (see Wolinsky, Mosely, & Coe, 1986) yielded only zero-order estimates of the
aging, period, and cohort effects. The reason is that those preliminary
analyses did not employ regression techniques to adjust the cell means
for the full panoply of predisposing, enabling, and need characteristics
contained in the behavioral model (see Andersen, 1968). When the
regression-based cohort analytic techniques were used to obtain more
pristine estimates of the net effects of aging, period, and cohort on
health and health behavior, however, no aging effects were detected
for either of the measures of physician use. Indeed, the only aging
effect detected in the regression-based cohort analysis involved limited activity owing to health reasons, a relationship consistently reported in the literature (see Cornoni-Huntley et al., 1985). Thus, the
regression-based cohort analysis results are entirely consistent with
those reported by Shapiro and Tate (1989), which also employed
multiple-regression techniques to adjust the data for differences in
sex, educational attainment, perceived health status, the taking of bed
disability days, and prior physician contact. Accordingly, the external
validity of the present study is markedly enhanced.

Effects of Age, Period, and Cohort
on Structural Relationships

Table 6.3 contains a summary of the aging, period, and cohort effects
on the effects of the predisposing, enabling, and need characteristics
on the dependent variables. As such, this table identifies those structural relationships that changed as the cohorts aged and passed
through different periods, as well as across cohorts at the same point.
These were detected by first estimating the behavioral model (see
Andersen, 1968) separately within each cell of the standard cohort
tables for each of the 10 dependent variables. The partial, unstandardized regression coefficients obtained were then used as the cell values
for the construction of a new set of 156 cohort tables. These tables
were then visually and statistically inspected for any aging, period, or
cohort changes in the partial, unstandardized regression coefficients.

Before proceeding to a review of the results shown in Table 6.3, three general comments warrant brief mention here. First, although 156 tables were examined, only 7 contained structural relationships that were altered by either age, period, or cohort effects. Second, no cohort effects were detected for any of these 7 structural relationships. Third, only 2 of the 7 structural relationships were affected by a period effect. When taken together, this indicates that the structural relationships between the predisposing, enabling, and need characteristics, and health and health behavior, are remarkably stable. Indeed, they are for the most part invariant as the cohorts age and pass through different historical periods, as well as between cohorts at the same point.

Because of the remarkable stability of the structural relationships overall, the review of the results shown in Table 6.3 is necessarily brief. For the most part, the changes in the structural relationships involve aging effects. Moreover, these aging effects reflect modest increases as the cohorts age, but only for the younger cohorts. This suggests that the changes result from either anticipatory role socialization (see Rosow, 1985), or the acceptance of the inevitability or normative aspects of poor health associated with being elderly (see Ferraro, 1980; Fillenbaum, 1979), or both. Each of these explanations is consistent with a pattern of change that is resolved by transition to elderly status, which most commonly occurs at or about retirement age. Accordingly, these aging effects are most likely the result of social aging, inasmuch as the changes in the structural relationships stabilize after the retirement threshold is crossed.

Caveats On Limitations of Data

Although the reconciliation of the two cohort analytic techniques enhances both the internal and external validity of the study, the HIS data are not without their own limitations. Indeed, three caveats concerning these data warrant special attention here. The first is that these analyses are based on synthetic (or cross-sequential) longitudinal data. That is, a sequence of representative cross-sectional samples of each cohort is drawn over time rather than tracking the same sample (i.e., panel) of each cohort as it ages. As a result, intraindividual change cannot be assessed in these analyses. Instead, inferences about intraindividual change are made based on the interindividual change that is observed. This problem, however, is minimized by the external validity provided by the consistency of these results with those obtained from the MLSA (see Mossey & Shapiro, 1985;

Table 6.3 Summary of Aging, Period, and Cohort Effects on Effects of Predisposing, Enabling, and Need Characteristics on Dependent Variables

Affected relationship	Aging effect	Period effect	Cohort effect
Effect of income on dental contact rates	None	Consistent increase	None
Effect of limited activity on physician contact rates	None	None	None
Effect of limited activity on physician visits	None	None	None
Effect of perceived health on the taking of restricted activity days	Slow increase limited to the younger cohorts	None	None
Effect of perceived health on the taking of bed disability days	Slow increase limited to the younger cohorts	None	None
Effect of perceived health on hospital contact rates	Increase limited to the younger cohorts	None	None

Effect of being a woman on perceived health	Decline and elimination of the differential by the onset of retirement	None	None
Effect of living alone on perceived health	Increase that stabilizes by retirement	None	None
Effect of family income on perceived health	None	Consistent increase for age-groups under 80	None

Mossey et al., 1981; Roos & Shapiro, 1981; Shapiro & Tate, 1989), which is indeed a panel analysis.

The second caveat concerns measurement errors involving the indicators included in the analysis that tap the predisposing, enabling, need, and health services use characteristics. For example, the two dichotomous measures of need, perceived health and limited activity owing to health reasons, are not extremely sensitive (i.e., discriminating). Moreover, both are based on self-reports. There would clearly be advantages to having more detailed indices, such as symptom checklists and disease histories, or physician examinations and laboratory assessments. Incorporating measures of psychological distress or depression would be valuable as well. The measures of the use of health services are also rather primitive. Using the measures of physician use as examples, no indication exists of either the purpose of the visit, or by whom the visit was initiated. Reducing such measurement errors would enhance the robustness of the predictive models of health and health behavior.

Specification errors involving variables hypothesized to be part of the behavioral model (see Andersen, 1968) but not available for inclusion in these analyses is the third limitation of the HISs. Particularly absent here are measures of the extent and nature of health insurance (both public and private), the characteristics of the areal health care delivery system (especially including supply and pricing factors), and the health beliefs of the individual respondents. The limitations imposed by the absence of these factors, however, is minimized given three factors. First, Counte and colleagues (see Glandon, Counte, & Homan, 1989; Homan, Glandon, & Counte, 1989) have shown that elderly individuals are generally poorly informed about the nature of their health insurance coverage. This questions the validity of using such information based on self-reports even when it is available. Second, Wolinsky et al., (1989) have shown that the characteristics of the health care delivery system in the respondent's metropolitan area, whether measured at the general or ethnic-specific level, are not predictive of the use of health services. Thus, the absence of such measures is likely to be of little consequence. Third, Andersen (1968) has shown that general (i.e., non–disease-specific) health beliefs are fundamentally unrelated to the use of health services. Therefore, the absence of health beliefs is also likely to be of little consequence.

Accordingly, then, the limitations that arise from (a) the intraindividual assessment of change, and (b) model specification issues are relatively minor. This leaves only the measurement error issue to be addressed. Although the measurement error problem does affect the estimates obtained for the behavioral model, such measurement errors only minimally affects the estimation of aging, period, and cohort effects. The reason for this is that there are no plausible grounds on which to expect that the effects of age, period, and cohort are correlated with these measurement difficulties. Therefore, the estimates of these (i.e., aging, period, and cohort) effects is unbiased. As a result, confidence in the results obtained from these analyses is generally unaffected by the known limitations of the data.

DISCUSSION

As indicated at the beginning of this chapter, five critical issues emerged from these analyses that warrant further discussion. They include (a) the negligible effects of aging, (b) the modest effects of period, (c) the substantial cohort effect on dental contact rates, (d) increasing income barriers to dental care, and (e) the fact that need is the most discriminating predictor of the use of health services. Each issue is addressed in this section, with special attention being given to their implications for the direction of future research on the health and health behavior of elderly Americans.

Negligible Effects of Aging

Perhaps the most important finding to emerge from this study is the negligible effect that aging has on health and health behavior. This is especially apparent in the results obtained from the regression-based cohort analysis, in which the only unique aging effect observed involved limited activity owing to health reasons. Moreover, even when the zero-order results from the traditional cohort analysis are considered, the effects of aging are, at best, minimal. Thus, this finding is not an artifact of the new methodology. Two important implications stem from this. First, the absence of meaningful aging effects reflects the remarkable heterogeneity that exists regarding the health and health behavior of elderly Americans. As such, it underscores the long-standing call for the end of the latent homogeneity assumption discussed in detail in Chapter 2 (see also Kovar, 1977, 1986). That is, it can no longer be plausibly assumed that all elderly individuals will behave the same, or that uniform behavior will be observed within different age-grades.

The second implication stems from the first. As indicated in Chapter 2 (see also Maddox & Lawton, 1988), age has limited utility as a discriminating factor in the health and health behavior of older people. This has special relevance for statistical modeling. It underscores the need for multivariate approaches that emphasize the individuality of older adults. From the practical standpoint, this augers for more complex analyses in which age is no longer relied on as a primary method for "cutting-the-deck" (in an analysis of variance sense). Instead, those analyses must focus on the underlying social-psychological and structural processes that facilitate or impede an elderly individual's health and health behavior.

On the social psychological side, considerably more attention must be given to understanding the "black box" phenomenon. That is, what is it in the individual's personal makeup that allows him or her to tolerate, or not tolerate, various signs and symptoms, and subsequently decide to seek, or not seek, health services in response to them (see Mechanic, 1978). Although several different researchers have proposed schematics to explain this "black box" (see Antonovsky's [1979, 1987] discussion of the sense of coherence, Kobassa's [1979] conception of the hardiness factor, Mechanic's [1979a, 1979b, 1980, 1983] identification of the distress syndrome and its ties to introspection and body awareness, or Pearlin's [Pearlin & Schooler, 1978; Pearlin, Lieberman, Menaghan, & Mullan, 1981] focus on self-mastery), little agreement exists on the fundamental process involved. Indeed, the hallmark of this work is that the principals involved downplay the apparent convergent validity of the different constructs at the same time that they are unable to demonstrate any divergent validity. Nonetheless, the next generation of advances in understanding the health and health behavior of elderly Americans will likely emerge from this work (see Hansell, Sherman, & Mechanic, 1990; Mechanic, 1989a).

On the structural side, the nature of the areal health care delivery system and the individual's real and perceived access to it (including age, gender, fiscal, and cultural barriers) must receive increased attention. As Ward (1978) has cogently noted, the increasing cautiousness and fatalism of the elderly make it particularly difficult for them to navigate successfully the fragmented and bureaucratic terrain of the American health care delivery system. This suggests that further study of the encounters between patients and their primary care practitioners (see Waitzkin, 1989; West, 1984), especially those involving older adults (see Coe & Prendergast, 1985; Coe, Prendergast, &

Psathas, 1984), should prove rather fruitful. The benefit of these studies would be enhanced by considering the fit between the patient and provider in terms of ascribed status characteristics, like ethnicity, religion, social class, and other markers of structural solidarity (see Aguirre, Wolinsky, Keither, Niederhauer, & Fann, 1989). Although the potential for research along these lines to increase the robustness of models of health and health behavior is considerable, disappointingly few researchers are actively engaged in such efforts.

Ultimately, gerontological studies of health and health behavior must shift their focus away from age as the primary determinant, and concentrate on the underlying processes. Moreover, to identify those processes they must recognize the need to employ perspectives like the age-stratification approach that simultaneously consider and estimate the net effects of age, period, and cohort (see Riley, 1972, 1973, 1976, 1985, 1987; Riley, Foner, Moore, Hess & Roth, 1968; Riley, Foner, & Waring, 1988). Although this requires more complex conceptualizations and concomitant statistical analyses, no alternative exists. The accumulated evidence compellingly demonstrates that when pristine estimates of the net effects of age are obtained, age plays an inconsequential role in the health and health behavior of the elderly. Simply put, it is time to refocus attention on individuals and the social processes that impinge on them, and abandon the primitive reliance on aggregate classifications based on chronological age.

Modest Effects of Period

One class of social processes that impinge on individuals is the effect of changing times. Of particular interest here are period effects that reflect changes in either access to or reimbursement for health services. Two notable examples of such changes involve the measures of physician and hospital use. Although the period effects identified on these variables were somewhat modest, they were nonetheless palpable and attributable to changes in the supply and insurance mechanisms available to elderly Americans.

The period effects on the use of physicians' services reflect the seemingly schizophrenic goals of American health care policy during the last three decades. That is, in recent times health policy in this country has focused in a near-simultaneous fashion on expanding access to health care while controlling costs. Whether this condition is best explained by the traditionally myopic approach to health planning (see Rushing, 1985) or by the competing interests of elites vested with distinctive institutional loyalties (see Laumann & Knoke, 1987) is of little relevance. In the end, the message was to do more for a greater number of people while spending less.

That message is reflected in the period effects observed for the two measures of physician use. On the one hand, an increase in physician contact rates occurred for all age-groups over time. This is consistent with the reports of Aday and colleagues (see Aday, Andersen, & Fleming, 1980; Aday, Fleming, & Andersen, 1984) that access to health care, defined as having seen a physician at least once during the past 12 months, has steadily risen since the early 1970s. Conversely, among those with access there was a decline in the number of physician visits per person per year. This is consistent with several reports (see Eisenberg, 1986; Estes, 1988; Stoeckle, 1987, 1988) that document increasing constraints on both patient- and provider-initiated visits imposed by third-party insurers as a cost-containment mechanism.

The period effects observed for the measures of hospital use also reflect the changing nature of the reimbursement process. They are not, however, entirely consistent with the general expectations concerning the perverse incentives introduced by Medicare's PPS and its associated DRGs (see Fetter, Shin, Freeman, Averill, & Thompson, 1980). It has been widely assumed that although the introduction of DRGs would reduce average lengths of stay for hospital visits (a cost-containment goal), they would also increase the number of admissions as providers sought to compensate for the reduced and fixed payment schedule (see Wolinsky, 1988a). Therefore, accelerations were expected after DRGs were implemented in the trends observed throughout the 1950s, 1960s, and 1970s for rising numbers of admissions and declining lengths of stay (reflecting, again, the competing goals of expanding access and containing costs [see Rushing, 1985]).

As the results of the regression-based cohort analysis indicate, however, such a scenario was not fully observed. On the one hand, a substantial increase in hospital contact rates did occur between the early and mid-1980s. This is consistent with the anticipated effects of DRGs. Conversely, the number of hospital episodes among those with at least one admission was rather stable during the 1980s, after increasing during the 1970s. Although the number of nights spent in the hospital did decline during the 1980s, that decline showed no acceleration of the same trend observed for the decade of the 1970s. These results are not at all consistent with the expectations regarding the perverse incentives of the PPS. Accordingly, although the data do reveal period effects on the demand for hospital services, those effects are not solely the result of DRGs.

The detection of such period effects on the measures of physician and hospital use underscores the importance of the social and political context in which that behavior is embedded. This goes beyond the fact that failing to control simultaneously for period effects would have resulted in the misleading identification of aging effects, emphasizing further the value of comprehensive perspectives like the age-stratification approach (see Riley, 1972, 1973, 1976, 1985, 1987; Riley et al., 1968; Riley et al., 1988). Indeed, the identification of these period effects highlights the salience of historical factors too long ignored in the routine analysis of health and health behavior.

Substantial Cohort Effect on Dental Contact Rates

Another class of social processes that impinge on people are subsumed under the rubric of cohort effects. The most notable cohort effect observed in these data involved dental contact rates. Older cohorts having lower rates of dental contact were being replaced by younger cohorts having higher rates of dental contact. That is, although oral health behavior is a relatively stable trait over the life course of adults (see Kiyak, 1987) for which pattern formation occurs at early ages (see Kegeles, 1963), successive birth cohorts are socialized to dissimilar expectations (see Elder, 1974, 1975; Elder & Liker, 1982). Regarding oral health behavior, the expectations facing younger cohorts progressively increased. Accordingly, as older generations leave and younger ones enter the standard cohort table, dental contact rates rise appreciably.

Although less striking, similar cohort effects are found for three other variables. The taking of restricted activity days and the number of physician visits both exhibit increases associated with cohort succession. Younger cohorts appear to be more willing to respond to health problems by taking time off and going to see a physician. This is consistent with the general perception that older cohorts tend to be more stoic and accepting of their lot in life, perhaps relying less on the use of external coping mechanisms (see Elder, 1974, 1975; Elder & Liker, 1982). Similarly, the younger cohorts are more likely to have poorer perceptions of their health status than are their older counterparts, all other things being equal. This suggests that the root cause of the traditionally observed difference in health-status assessment between the young-old and the old-old (see Ferraro, 1980; Fillenbaum, 1979) is not due to age per se, but to the differential experiences associated with birth cohorts.

The detection of these cohort effects is important beyond their demonstration of the utility of the age-stratification perspective (see Riley, 1972, 1973, 1976, 1985, 1987; Riley et al., 1968; Riley et al., 1988), without which they would not have been observed. These cohort effects also underscore the importance of distinguishing between use of discretionary and nondiscretionary health services. That is, the largest cohort effects were found for the most discretionary health service (i.e., dentists' services), whereas no cohort effects were found for the least discretionary health service (i.e., hospitals' services). Among those health services of a mixed discretionary status, the observed cohort effects were rather modest.

This is precisely the pattern that one would expect. The potential for the life experiences of one's birth cohort to influence health and health behavior should crest in situations of individual choice, and ebb in situations where others are in decision-making positions. Moreover, inasmuch as the extent of insurance coverage for health services varies inversely with their discretionary nature, cohort effects on dental contact rates are least likely to have been eroded by public policy programs designed to achieve an equitable health care delivery system (see Wolinsky & Coe, 1984). This further accounts for the differential magnitude of the observed cohort effects.

Increasing Income Barriers to Dental Care

The most marked change observed on the effects of the predisposing, enabling, and need characteristics on the use of health services involved the effect of income on dental contact rates. Over time, real income barriers (i.e., adjusted for changes in the Consumer Price Index) between elderly Americans and dentists' services increased substantially. That is, the partial, unstandardized regression coefficient of income on dental contact became progressively and significantly larger over time for all age-groups. Indeed, as can be derived from Table 5.11, the increase in the magnitude of those regression coefficients between the early 1970s and the early 1980s (note that dental contact was not measured in the HISs during the mid-1980s) averaged 86%.

Such changes reflect important alterations in older adults' access to dental care (see Wolinsky & Arnold, 1989). Although dental care may seem to be a relatively unimportant health service (when compared with access to physician and hospital services), this is not the case among the elderly. Less than optimal oral health behavior increases the likelihood of gerodontic diseases, which increase the risk of edentulism (see Beck, 1984). Edentulism (especially when ill-fitting dentures result) increases the likelihood of disadvantageous dietary intake owing to the mechanical problems associated with biting and chewing (see Wolinsky et al., 1986). Poor dietary intake results in nutritional deficits, which in turn increase the risk of disease (see McIntosh, Shifflet, & Picou, 1989), especially given the reduced functional reserves of the elderly (see Cape, Coe, & Rossman, 1983). As these data (and others, see Chapter 2) have shown, health status is the major determinant of the use of health services. Thus, in the long run, oral health behavior is of considerable public policy import.

Moreover, these changes also suggest that access to other health services that are routinely not covered by insurance has declined as well. That is, at the more abstract level, dental contact can be considered as just one of many measures of discretionary and relatively uninsured health behavior. Therefore, it is plausible to assume that the effects of income on other health behaviors for which dental contact may be considered a proxy have also increased over time. If that is the case, and no apparent reason exists to suspect otherwise, then access to the entire panoply of discretionary and relatively uninsured health services (such as prevention, health maintenance, and home health care) has become less equitable as well. This would indicate the existence of rather widespread socioeconomic discrimination.

Need as the Most Discriminating Variable

The variable that emerged from these analyses as the most predictive of health behavior was need, as measured by perceived health status and limited activity owing to health reasons. This is not at all surprising inasmuch as the literature reviewed in Chapter 2 has consistently reached the same conclusion. There is less agreement, however, on what this means. According to Andersen and colleagues (see Aday & Andersen, 1981; Aday et al., 1980, 1984; Andersen, 1968; Andersen & Newman, 1973), this fact can be taken as an indication that the health care delivery system is equitable. They argue that equity exists when only medical need determines the use of health services (in addition to some vestiges of a relationship with age and sex, as proxies of biological need). In contrast, an inequitable system is said to exist if the use of health services is distributed on the basis of other factors, like race, income, or place of residence.

That interpretation, however, is not held by everyone. For example, Mechanic (1985) has argued that access to health care for the poor and elderly (two groups with considerable overlap) have been eroding since these data were collected, and that further losses can be expected to result from current budgetary constraints. Similarly, Berki et al., (1985) have shown with chilling starkness how the economic hardships of the early 1980s disenfranchised many of the unemployed and underemployed from traditional private and public health insurance programs. Using actuarial methods, Farley (1985) has estimated that 56 million Americans are now inadequately protected against the possibility of large medical bills (defined as 10% or more of their family income).

Aside from disagreements like these, which basically focus on deteriorating access associated with the economic downturn of the 1980s, Wolinsky, Coe, and Mosely (1987) and Mechanic (1979c, 1989a) raise more telling objections to the equity interpretation advanced by Andersen and colleagues (see Aday & Andersen, 1981; Aday et al., 1980, 1984; Andersen, 1968; Andersen & Newman, 1973). The tack taken by Wolinsky and colleagues is that although (a) the need characteristics are the primary determinants of the use of health services, and (b) the effects of the predisposing and enabling characteristics are generally marginal, less than 25% of the variance in the use of health services is explained. Because most of the variance remains unexplained, and assuming that the use of health services is not a random phenomenon, they argue that it is premature to declare the health care delivery system to be equitable. That is, while the underlying causes of health behavior remain unknown, it is inappropriate to assume that those unknown causes are unrelated to anything except need.

Mechanic (1979c, 1989a) takes a more devastating philosophical position. He argues that what commonly passes for measures of need are more accurate reflections of health behavior. That is, the traditional measures of need actually reflect more of the individual's perception of symptoms, pattern recognition of the conditions that they represent, and behavioral response to those health problems than they do to the health problems themselves. Two problems ultimately result from this compounded measurement error. First, health is not adequately represented in these models. Second, given the contamination of the measures of health status with health behavior, the empirical relationships between need and the use of health services are overestimated. Therefore, it is unwarranted to use these overestimates as a basis for declaring equity in the health care delivery system.

When taken together, (a) the fact that need is the most discriminating predictor of the use of health services, and (b) the controversy surrounding the interpretation of that relationship suggest that a new direction in health and health behavior studies is warranted. Perhaps it is time to roll back the focus in causal models from the use of health services to the need characteristics. That is, virtually all work in this area seeks to explain the use of health services. It would be rather fruitful at this point to shift attention toward understanding the perception, recognition, and behavioral response of individuals to deviations in their physical, social, and psychological functioning. Such an approach has special appeal inasmuch as it would involve parallel efforts (offering considerable potential for efficiency and cross-fertilization) with ongoing work aimed at understanding the "black box" described earlier (see Antonovsky, 1979, 1987; Kobassa, 1979; Mechanic, 1978, 1979a, 1979b, 1979c, 1980, 1983; Pearlin, 1978; Pearlin et al., 1981). Here, however, the focus would be on understanding the causal nexus of self-assessed health status.

RESTRUCTURING THE AMERICAN HEALTH CARE DELIVERY SYSTEM: AN IMMODEST PROPOSAL

Based on the review of the extant literature and the analyses presented earlier, a fundamental restructuring of the American health care delivery system seems warranted. Such a statement flies in the face of the long-standing reliance on the "risk factor approach" for the allocation of health care benefits and the tradition of "pragmatic incrementalism," both of which are deeply embedded in American public policy (see Binstock, 1985). Indeed, it has been forcefully argued that the likelihood of such momentous change is not great (see Estes & Newcomer, 1983). Nonetheless, the time has come to abandon such concerns and consider instead alternative structures that more fully address the limitations of the current system (see Davis, 1985).

The underlying purpose of the admittedly immodest proposal presented here is to bring about a system that is not only more equitable in terms of access to an expanded array of needed health services but is also more likely to constrain costs. This proposal is based on five precepts, including (a) a shift from age-based to need-based criteria, (b) expanded coverage, (c) the encouragement of prevention as well as health promotion and maintenance, (d) the introduction of a universal and mandatory national health insurance program for all age-groups, and (e) the reliance on primary care physicians as the cornerstones and gatekeepers of the new system. Although each precept is only briefly discussed in rather general terms subsequently, the rationale should be sufficiently clear to facilitate its discussion and an assessment of its merits.

Shift From Age-Based to Need-Based Criteria

The two most important findings to emerge from this study are that age (per se) is fundamentally unrelated to the use of health services, and that need (i.e., health status) is the most discriminating factor in their prediction. Yet, in the current social welfare system (i.e., Social Security and Medicare), chronological age is the basic criterion for service eligibility. Although historical factors may explain why this mismatch between the cause of and eligibility for the use of health services came into being (such as with the enactment of the Social Security legislation that opted for an absolute rather than a relative chronological age marker, see Chapter 2), they can no longer be used to justify its continued existence. Given the remarkable evidence for the heterogeneity of the health and health behavior of the elderly, the time for a need-based health care policy has come.

To be sure, this is not a novel precept. Perhaps the most eloquent pleas in this regard have come from Neugarten (1974, 1979, 1982). Besides the simple fact that age-based criteria are not relevant, she argues that they have created an increased perception of the "graying of the budget." That is a dangerous situation because (Neugarten, 1982):

> If age-based rather than need-based legislation continues, those of us who consider ourselves advocates for older people may inadvertently be creating age discrimination at the very same time we decry it. Policies and programs aimed at "the old," while they may have been intended to compensate for inequity and disadvantage, may have the unintended effect of adding to age segregation, of reinforcing the misperception of "the old" as a problem group, and of stigmatizing rather than liberating older people from the negative effects of the label, "old." (p. 27)

Indeed, Binstock (1985) has argued that the continued reliance on age-based criteria in the 1980s has increased the occurrence of "tabloid thinking" in which the elderly are portrayed as the root cause of the current federal budgetary crisis. A noteworthy example of this phenomenon is Callahan's (1987) proposal for an age-based (i.e., age 75) cut-off for coverage of expensive health care procedures by Medicare.

What are the major obstacles confronting a shift to need-based criteria? Although Neugarten (1982) focuses primarily on political, social, and economic factors, she ignores the most pragmatic issues. How will the need for health services (based on health status) be assessed, who will make those assessments, and for how long will such assessments be in force? To be sure, one of the most positive aspects of age-based criteria is their ease of administration. The shift to need-based criteria will require more thoughtful and repetitive assessments, inasmuch as eligibility will likely be determined on an episodic or conditional basis rather than on a permanent basis. These problems, however, are not insurmountable and are addressed later in the context of the fifth precept.

Expanded Service Coverage

Another important finding to emerge from this study was the increasing socioeconomic barrier between older adults and their access to discretionary health services that are not routinely covered by insurance. The current health care delivery system has progressively become more inequitable in this regard. These inequities are compounded by the fact that other needed but uninsured social and otherwise nonmedical services that are pertinent to achieving and maintaining good health (see Cantor & Little, 1985) are also differentially distributed on the basis of socioeconomic status. This not only creates and maintains a two-tiered system of health care (one for the self-sufficient and another for the dependent), it also makes that system less efficient and effective. That is, to the extent that the more discretionary and routinely uninsured health services, in conjunction with the social and other nonmedical services facilitate prevention, health promotion and maintenance, and early detection, any access barriers to them result in higher costs and less desirable outcomes.

Accordingly, it would seem both prudent and morally appropriate to expand the range of services covered under the new health care delivery system. Exactly what additional services, however, ought be included? At a minimum that list should contain dental services, institutional and noninstitutional long-term care, in-home services for more acute problems, and respite care (especially for the friends, neighbors, and family members currently providing the bulk of informal services to the elderly; see Brody, 1981, 1985; Cantor, 1979).

Perhaps more important than the inclusion of such services under the coverage umbrella, however, is some provision for their integration and coordination. That is, as Kane and Kane (1976), Lowy

(1979), and Tobin (1977) have noted, once access has been obtained, it is the judicious selection of these services that becomes crucial. Ward's (1978) observation that the increasing cautiousness and fatalism of the elderly makes it particularly difficult for them to negotiate the fragmented and bureaucratic terrain of the health care delivery system serves only to underscore this problem.

Although no ready solutions are available to this integration and coordination dilemma, the advent of Social and Health Maintenance Organizations (SHMOs) (see Diamond & Berman, 1979) in the 1980s may serve as a starting point. Basically, the logic of SHMOs is to expand the health maintenance organization (HMO) (see Luft, 1981) concept by including social and other nonmedical services under the managed care approach. In a managed care setting, the delivery system (i.e., the SHMO), acting as a fiduciary agent (see Parsons, 1951, 1975) for the enrolled individual, is responsible both for providing and coordinating any health and social services that are needed. This provides the elderly individual with both a gateway to and guide through the rapidly growing maze of social services (see Cantor & Little, 1985).

SHMOs, however, are not the ultimate answer. Like the HMOs from which they sprang, SHMOs are most viable in metropolitan areas that can support their break-even requirements of having 50,000 or more enrollees in relatively close proximity (see Luft, 1981). As of yet, little evidence exists of their efficiency and effectiveness. Nonetheless, the thought of a managed health and social care system in which the provider assumes responsibility for the integration and coordination of services has considerable appeal.

Prevention, and Health Promotion and Maintenance

Current health care policy in the United States is consistent with the medical model and its commitment to germ theory (see Twaddle & Hessler, 1987; Wolinsky, 1988a). As such, it focuses almost exclusively on combating disease. Indeed, 93.6% of all health care dollars are expended for medical care, and an additional 3.5% go toward research and construction. That leaves only 2.9% for public health activities (see National Association for Public Health Policy, 1989). As Dubos (1959) has written, this is analogous to the futile and never-ending search for "magic bullets."

The value of that search has come under even more severe criticism in recent years (see Levine, Feldman, & Elinson, 1983; McKeown, 1976; McKinlay & McKinlay, 1977; McKinlay, McKinlay, & Beaglehole, 1989). Mounting evidence now demonstrates that the increases in the health of the population that have occurred during the past three decades have relatively little to do with medical care per se. Rather, changes in personal health behavior and environmental quality account for the gains that have been made (see Kasl, 1986). These facts notwithstanding, funding for public health endeavors has remained relatively stable.

This rather ironic dilemma of supporting ineffective medical care instead of effective public health intervention has special implications for the elderly. On the one hand, the primary causes of death and disability for the elderly are preventable (see Verbrugge, 1984). Conversely, these same health problems are not well addressed by medical care (see Cape, et al., 1983). Therefore, it would seem prudent to encourage those traditionally more public health-oriented activities (such as prevention, and health promotion and maintenance) that are effective at reducing the risk for, adverse effects of, and recovery from the major "killer" and "limiting" diseases facing the elderly (see Marshall & Graham, 1986; Ostfeld, 1986; Whisnant, 1984). Moreover, given the considerable potential for cost-containment associated with such activities, their encouragment has pragmatic virtues as well (see Weinstein & Stason, 1985). In addition, such an approach would be entirely consistent with the notion of "individual responsibility" that permeates American health care policy (see Fox, 1987).

Accordingly, the third precept in this rather immodest proposal for restructuring the American health care delivery system involves encouraging prevention, and health promotion and maintenance. The primary method of encouraging such behavior is by providing fiscal incentives to the elderly. Those incentives would involve first-dollar, complete reimbursement without any direct billing to the user. That is, the use of physician and nonphysician providers for prevention, and health maintenance and promotion services would be fully covered, with no deductibles or copayments. Moreover, bills for such services would be submitted directly to the insurance fund by the provider. This would permit the desired service consumption without any out-of-pocket costs by the elderly individual, and without his or her having to seek reimbursement from the insurance fund. As in HMOs (see Luft, 1981), this should serve as a powerful stimulant for such desired use.

Universal, Mandatory National Health Insurance

The fourth precept of this immodest proposal for restructuring the American health care delivery system is that it must involve a universal, mandatory national health insurance (NHI) program for all age-groups. As Fuchs (1974) wrote more than a decade and a half ago, three important benefits accrue from such an approach. First, it is the most opportune method for integrating the poor, both working and nonworking, into the same health care delivery system that covers the bulk of society (see also Petersen, 1987). As such, a universal, mandatory NHI would eliminate the two-tiered (or multitiered, see Wolinsky, 1988a) aspects of the system currently in place. At best, those tiers can be described as separate but not equal (see Salloway, 1982). Therefore, if access to health care is indeed a fundamental right of all Americans (see Fox, 1987), then a universal, mandatory NHI is a straightforward method of securing that platitude.

Second, a universal, mandatory NHI allows national standards to be established, both in terms of service benefits and administrative structures (see Fuchs, 1974). National standards for service benefits are more consistent with a fundamental rights argument (see Fox, 1987) than are locally determined coverage schedules. Moreover, reliance on national standards facilitates more rapid readjustment of coverage issues as new medical technologies and treatment regimens come on line, and as existing ones are altered. Similarly, the reliance on national standards also facilitates the implementation of changes in the reimbursement process. Such a plan permits the changes described earlier to be phased in more gradually.

The third benefit of such a universal, mandatory NHI is derived from the first two. Simply put, there is considerable symbolic value to this approach (see Fuchs, 1984). Because all Americans would be involved, such a plan would focus attention on serving the nation rather than reaching out to any one particular entitlement group. As a result, issues like the "graying of the budget" (see Neugarten, 1974, 1979, 1982) and other examples of "tabloid thinking" (see Binstock, 1985), which pit one segment of society against another (or the middle), would disappear. Instead, the costs (both real and perceived) of the new system would be consensually viewed as part of the infrastructure necessary to support national goals and objectives.

Primary Care Physicians as Cornerstones and Gatekeepers

The final precept involves designating primary care physicians as the cornerstones and gatekeepers of the new health care delivery system. In that role, primary care physicians would have the authority and responsibility to assess the needs of and coordinate the care (both medical and nonmedical) for their patients. This would enhance the coordination and continuity of care that is especially critical in treating elderly patients (see Cape et al., 1983). It would also provide considerable opportunity to increase the appropriate and decrease the inappropriate use of medical specialists.

Such an approach rests on two important assumptions. The first is that individuals will seek out primary care physicians and comply with their recommendations. A pair of fiscal incentives currently employed in the health care delivery system will facilitate such behavior (see Eisenberg, 1986; Luft, 1981). One involves eliminating all out-of-pocket costs for visits to primary care physicians. The other involves eliminating all out-of-pocket costs for services provided by medical specialists and other providers on referral from the primary care physician. When taken together, these fiscal incentives will effectively influence health behavior, providing that (at least on an annual basis) individuals have free choice of their primary care physicians (see Mechanic, 1989b; Sammons, 1989).

The second important assumption on which such an approach rests is that primary care physicians will behave as fiduciary agents for their patients while maintaining their societal responsibilities as a service profession (see Freidson, 1970a, 1970b, 1980, 1986; Parsons, 1951, 1975). Although such behavior is entirely consistent with traditional image of doctoring contained in the Hippocratic Oath and the Prayer of Maimonides, critics have questioned whether changing times in the health care industry have eroded such commitments and practices (see Hafferty, 1988; Light & Levine, 1988; Stoeckle, 1988; Wolinsky, 1988b). Regardless of whether any erosion has occurred, fiscal incentives can be brought to bear on primary care physicians to encourage such behavior.

Basically, these fiscal incentives would involve a shift to a capitation-based payment system. Primary care physicians would receive a flat annual budget for providing and coordinating all of the health (both medical and nonmedical) care needed by their panel of patients. This budget would be divided into a fixed capitation account for the primary care physicians' services, and a reserve account for all those services provided by others on his or her referral. Unexpended funds in the reserve accounts for different patients of the same primary care physician could be commingled to offset losses incurred as a result of catastrophic costs, or, rolled over into the next capitation period (essentially returning any "profits" to the benefit of the patient panel). Such an incentive structure would go a long way toward

eliminating the perverse incentives of the current system while encouraging cost-containment (see Wolinsky, 1988a).

Epilogue

Each of the five precepts on which the proposed restructuring of the
American health care delivery system is based have only been briefly
described here. Much remains to be done to flesh out the details. In
addition, a careful projection of the associated costs needs to be made.
Nonetheless, the intent of the admittedly immodest proposal is clear.
The time has come to address the limitations of the current health
care delivery system fully, especially as they apply to the elderly. In
addressing those needs, there must be a thoughtful stewardship of
available resources. The proposal presented here should stimulate a
discussion of the problems and options available to achieve those
goals.

REFERENCES

Aday, L. A., & Andersen, R. M. (1981). Equity of access to medical care: A
    conceptual and empirical overview. *Medical Care, 19,* S4–S27.
Aday, L. A., Andersen, R. M., & Fleming, G. V. (1980). *Health care in the U.S.:
    Equitable for whom?* Beverly Hills: Sage Publications.
Aday, L. A., Fleming, G. V., & Andersen, R. M. (1984). *Access to medical care in the
    U.S.: Who has it, who doesn't.* Chicago: Pluribus Press.
Aguirre, B. E., Wolinsky, F. D., Keith, V. M., Niederhauer, J., & Fann, L. J. (1989).
    Occupational prestige in the health care delivery system. *Journal of Health and
    Social Behavior, 30,* 315–329.
Andersen, R. M. (1968). *A behavioral model of families' use of health services.* Chicago:
    Center for Health Administration Studies.
Andersen, R. M., & Newman, J. F. (1973). Societal and individual determinants of
    medical care utilization in the U.S. *Milbank Memorial Fund Quarterly, 51,* 95–
    124.
Antonovsky, A. (1979). *Health, stress, and coping: New perspectives on mental and
    physical well-being.* San Francisco: Jossey-Bass.
Antonovsky, A. (1987). *Unraveling the mystery of health: How people manage stress and
    stay well.* San Francisco: Jossey-Bass.
Beck, J. D. (1984). The epidemiology of dental diseases in the elderly. *Gerodontology,*
    3:5–15.
Berki, S., Wyszewianski, L., Lichtenstein, R., Gimotty, P., Bowlyow, J., Papke, E.,
    Smith, T., Crane, S., & Bromberg, J. (1985). Health insurance coverage of the
    unemployed. *Medical Care, 23,* 847–854.
Binstock, R. H. (1985). The oldest old: A fresh perspective or compassionate ageism
    revisited. *Milbank Memorial Fund Quarterly, 63,* 420–451.

Brody, E. M. (1981). Women in the middle and family help to older people. *The Gerontologist, 21*, 471–480.

Brody, E. M. (1985). Parent care as normative family stress. *The Gerontologist, 25*, 19–29.

Callahan, D. (1987). *Setting limits: Medical goals in an aging society.* New York: Simon & Schuster.

Cantor, M. (1979). Neighbors and friends: An overlooked resource in the informal support system. *Research on Aging, 1*, 434–463.

Cantor, M., & Little, V. (1985). Aging and social care. In R. Binstock & E. Shanas (Eds.), *Aging and the social sciences* (2nd ed.) (pp. 746–782). New York: Van Nostrand Reinhold.

Cape, R. T., Coe, R. M., & Rossman, I. (Eds.). (1983). *Fundamentals of geriatric medicine.* New York: Raven Press.

Coe, R. M., & Prendergast, C. (1985). The formation of coalitions: Interactive strategies in triads. *Sociology of Health and Illness, 7*, 236–247.

Coe, R. M., Prendergast, C., & Psathas, G. (1984). Strategies for obtaining compliance with medical regimens. *Journal of the American Geriatrics Society, 32*, 589–593.

Cornoni-Huntley, J. C., Foley, D. J., White, L. R., Suzman, R., Berkman, L. F., Evans, D. A., & Wallace, R. B. (1985). Epidemiology of disability in the oldest old: Methodologic issues and preliminary findings. *Milbank Memorial Fund Quarterly,* 63:350–376.

Davis, K. (1985). Health care policies and the aged: Observations from the United States. In R. Binstock & E. Shanas (Eds.). *Handbook of aging and the social sciences* (2nd ed.) (pp. 728–744). New York: Van Nostrand Reinhold.

Department of Health and Human Services. (1975). *The National Health Interview Survey procedure, 1957–1974* (DHHS Publication No. 75-1311). Washington, DC: Government Printing Office.

Department of Health and Human Services. (1985). *The National Health Interview Survey design, 1973–1984* (DHHS Publication No. 85-1320). Washington, DC: Government Printing Office.

Diamond, L., & Berman, D. (1979). *The social health maintenance organization: A single entry, prepaid, long-term care delivery system.* Brandeis University, Boston.

Dubos, R. (1959). *The mirage of health.* New York: Doubleday & Co.

Eisenberg, J. M. (1986). *Doctors' decisions and the cost of medical care.* Ann Arbor: Health Administration Press.

Elder, G. H. (1974). *Children of the Great Depression.* Chicago: University of Chicago Press.

Elder, G. H. (1975). Age differentiation and the life course. *Annual Review of Sociology, 1*, 165–190.

Elder, G. H., & Liker, J. K. (1982). Hard times in women's lives: Historical influences across 40 years. *American Journal of Sociology, 88*, 241–269.

Estes, C. L. (1988). *Organizational and community responses to medicare policy: Consequences for health and social services for the elderly* (vol. 1). San Francisco: Institute for Health and Aging.

Estes, C. L., & Newcomer, R. J. (1983). *Fiscal austerity and aging: Shifting government responsibility for the elderly.* Beverly Hills: Sage Publications.

Farley, P. J. (1985). Who are the underinsured? *Milbank Memorial Fund Quarterly, 63*, 476–503.

Ferraro, K. R. (1980). Self-ratings of health among the old and the old-old. *Journal of Health and Social Behavior, 21,* 377–382.

Fetter, R. B., Shin, Y., Freeman, J. L., Averill, R. F., & Thomspon, J. (1980). Case mix definition by diagnostic related groups. *Medical Care, 18,* S1–S136.

Fillenbaum, G. G. (1979). Social context and self-assessments of health among the elderly. *Journal of Health and Social Behavior, 20,* 45–51.

Fox, D. M. (1987). AIDs and the American health polity: The history and prospects of a crisis in authority. *The Milbank Quarterly, 64,* S7–S33.

Freidson, E. (1970a). *The profession of medicine: A study in the sociology of applied knowledge.* New York: Dodd, Mead.

Freidson, E. (1970b). *Professional dominance: The social structure of medical care.* New York: Atherton Press.

Freidson, E. (1980). *Doctoring together: A study of professional control.* Chicago: University of Chicago Press.

Freidson, E. (1986). *Professional powers: A study of the institutionalization of formal knowledge.* Chicago: University of Chicago Press.

Fuchs, V. R. (1974). *Who shall live? Health, economics, and social change.* New York: Basic Books.

Glandon, G. L., Counte, M. A., & Homan, R. (1989). *The elderly's knowledge of medicare coverage* (Report). Rush-Presbyterian-St. Luke's Medical Center, Chicago.

Glenn, N. D. (1976). Cohort analysts' futile quest: Statistical attempts to separate age, period, and cohort effects. *American Sociological Review, 41,* 900–904.

Glenn, N. D. (1977). *Cohort analysis.* Beverly Hills: Sage Publications.

Glenn, N. D. (1989). A flawed approach to solving the identification problem in the estimation of mobility effect models: A comment on Brody and McRae. *Social Forces, 67,* 789–795.

Hafferty, F. W. (1988). Theories at the crossroads: A discussion of evolving views on medicine as a profession. *The Milbank Quarterly, 66,* S202–225.

Hansell, S., Sherman, S., & Mechanic, D. (in press) Body awareness and the use of health services among the elderly. *Journal of Gerontology.*

Homan, R., Glandon, G. L., & Counte, M. A. (1989). Perceived risk: The link to plan selection and future utilization. *Journal of Risk and Insurance, 56,* 67–82.

Kane, R., & Kane, R. (1976). *Long-term care in six countries: Implications for the U.S* (DHEW Publication No. 76-1207). Washington, DC: Government Printing Office.

Kasl, S. B. (1986). The detection and modification of psychosocial and behavioral risk factors. In L. Aiken & D. Mechanic (Eds.), *Applications of social science to clinical medicine and health policy* (pp. 359–391). New Brunswick: Rutgers University Press.

Kegeles, S. S. (1963). Why people seek dental care: A test of a conceptual framework. *Journal of Health and Human Behavior, 4,* 166–175.

Kiyak, A. (1987). An exploratory model of older persons' use of dental services: Implications for health policy. *Medical Care, 25,* 936–951.

Kobassa, S. (1979). Stressful life events, personality, and health. *Journal of Personality and Social Psychology, 37,* 1–11.

Kovar, M. G. (1977). Health of the elderly and use of health services. *Public Health Reports, 92,* 9–19.

Kovar, M. G. (1986). Expenditures for medical care of elderly people living in the community in 1980. *The Milbank Quarterly, 64,* 100–132.

Laumann, E. O., & Knoke, D. (1987). *The organizational state: Social choice in national policy domains.* Madison: University of Wisconsin Press.

Levine, S., Feldman, J., & Elinson, J. (1983). Does medical care do any good? In D. Mechanic (Ed.), *Handbook of health, health care, and the health professions* (pp. 321–349). New York: Free Press.

Light, D., & Levine, S. (1988). The changing character of the medical profession: A theoretical overview. *The Milbank Quarterly, 66,* S10–S32.

Lowy, L. (1979). *Social work with the aging: The challenge and promise of the later years.* New York: Harper & Row.

Luft, H. S. (1981). *Health maintenance organizations: Dimensions of performance.* New York: John Wiley & Sons.

Maddox, G. L., & Lawton, M. P. (1988). Introduction. *Annual Review of Gerontology and Geriatrics, 8,* ix–xiii.

Manton, K. G., & Soldo, B. J. (1985). Dynamics of health changes in the oldest old: New perspectives and evidence. *Milbank Memorial Fund Quarterly, 63,* 206–285.

Marshall, J., & Graham, S. (1986). Cancer. In L. Aiken & Mechanic, D. (Eds.), *Applications of social science to clinical medicine and health policy* (pp. 157–174). New Brunswick: Rutgers University Press.

McIntosh, W. A., Shifflet, P. A., & Picou, S. J. (1989). Social support, stressful events, strain, dietary intake, and the elderly. *Medical Care, 27,* 140–153.

McKeown, T. (1976). *The role of medicine: Dream, mirage, or nemesis?* London: Nuffield Provincial Hospitals Trust.

McKinlay, J. B., & McKinlay, S. (1977). The questionable effect of medical measures on the decline of mortality in the United States in the twentieth century. *Milbank Memorial Fund Quarterly, 55,* 405–428.

McKinlay, J. B., McKinlay, S., & Beaglehole, R. (1989). Trends in death and disease and the contribution of medical measures. In H. Freeman & S. Levine, (Eds.), *Handbook of medical sociology* (4th ed.) (pp. 14–43). Englewood Cliffs, NJ: Prentice Hall.

Mechanic, D. (1978). *Medical sociology: A comprehensive text* (2nd ed.). New York: Free Press.

Mechanic, D. (1979a). Correlates of psychological distress among young adults: A theoretical hypothesis and results from a 16-year follow-up study. *Archives of General Psychiatry, 36,* 1233–1239.

Mechanic, D. (1979b). The stability of health and illness behavior: Results from a 16-year follow-up. *American Journal of Public Health, 69,* 1142–1145.

Mechanic, D. (1979c). Correlates of physician utilization: Why do major multivariate studies of physician utilization find trivial psychosocial effects? *Journal of Health and Social Behavior, 20,* 387–396.

Mechanic, D. (1980). The experience and reporting of common physical complaints. *Journal of Health and Social Behavior, 21,* 146–155.

Mechanic, D. (1983). The experience and expression of distress: The study of illness behavior and medical utilization. In D. Mechanic (Ed.), *Handbook of health, health care, and health professions* (pp. 174–201). New York: Free Press.

Mechanic, D. (1985). Cost containment and the quality of medical care: Rationing strategies in an era of constrained resources. *Milbank Memorial Fund Quarterly, 63,* 453–475.

Mechanic, D. (1989a). Medical sociology: Some tensions among theory, method, and substance. *Journal of Health and Social Behavior, 30,* 147–160.

Mechanic, D. (1989b). Consumer choice among health insurance options. *Health Affairs, 8,* 138–148.

Mossey, J. M., Havens, B., Roos, N. P., & Roos, L. (1981). The Manitoba Longitudinal Study on Aging: Description and methods. *The Gerontologist, 21,* 551–559.

Mossey, J. M., & Shapiro, E. (1985). Physician use by the elderly over an eight-year period. *American Journal of Public Health, 75,* 1333–1337.

National Association for Public Health Policy. (1989). *Put prevention first!* Burlington, VT: National Association for Public Health Policy.

Neugarten, B. L. (1974). Age groups in American society and the rise of the young old. *Annals of the American Academy of Political and Social Science, 415,* 187–198.

Neugarten, B. L. (1979). Age or need entitlement. In J. Hubbard (Ed.), *Aging: Agenda for the eighties* (pp. 1–13). Washington, DC: Government Research Corporation.

Neugarten, B. L. (1982). Policy for the 1980s: Age or Need Entitlement? In B. L. Neugarten (Ed.), *Age or need?* (pp. 1–11). Beverly Hills: Sage Publications.

Ostfeld, A. M. (1986). Cardiovascular disease. In L. Aiken & D. Mechanic (Eds.), *Applications of social science to clinical medicine and health policy* (pp. 129–156). New Brunswick: Rutgers University Press.

Palmore, E. (1978). When can age, period, and cohort be separated? *Social Forces, 57,* 285–295.

Parsons, T. (1951). *The social system.* New York: Free Press.

Parsons, T. (1975). The sick role and the role of the physician reconsidered. *Milbank Memorial Fund Quarterly, 53,* 257–278.

Pearlin, L. I., Lieberman, M. A. Menaghan, E. G., & Mullan, J. T. (1981). The stress process. *Journal of Health and Social Behavior, 22,* 337–357.

Pearlin, L. I., & Schooler, C. (1978). The structure of coping. *Journal of Health and Social Behavior, 19,* 2–21

Petersen, W. (1987). Politics and the measurement of ethnicity. In W. Alonso & P. Starr (eds.), *The politics of numbers* (pp. 187–212). New York: Russell Sage.

Riley, M. W. (1972). The succession of cohorts. In M. Riley, M. Johnson, & A. Foner (eds.), *Aging and society: A sociology of age stratification* (Vol. 3) (pp. 515–582). New York: Russell Sage.

Riley, M. W. (1973). Aging and cohort succession: Interpretations and misinterpretations. *Public Opinion Quarterly, 37,* 35–49.

Riley, M. W. (1976). Age strata in social systems. In R. Binstock & E. Shanas (Eds.), *Handbook of aging and the social sciences* (pp. 314–369). New York: Van Nostrand Reinhold.

Riley, M. W. (1985). Age strata in social systems. In R. Binstock & E. Shanas (Eds.), *Handbook of aging and the social sciences* (2nd ed.) (pp. 369–414). New York: Van Nostrand Reinhold.

Riley, M. W. (1987). On the significance of age in sociology. *American Sociological Review, 52,* 1–14.

Riley, M. W., Foner, A., Moore, M. E., Hess, B. B., & Roth, B. K. (1968). *Aging and society: An inventory of research findings* (Vol. 1). New York: Russell Sage.

Riley, M. W., Foner, A., & Waring, J. (1988). Sociology of age. In N. J. Smelser (Ed.), *Handbook of sociology* (pp. 243–290). Newbury Park, CA: Sage Publications.

Roos, N. P., & Shapiro, E. (1981). The Manitoba Longitudinal Study on Aging: Preliminary findings on health care utilization by the elderly. *Medical Care, 19,* 644–656.

Rosow, I. (1985). Status and role change through the life cycle. In R. Binstock & E. Shanas (Eds.), *Handbook of aging and the social sciences* (2nd ed.) (pp. 62–93). New York: Van Nostrand Reinhold.

Rushing, W. (1985). The supply of physicians and expenditures for health services with implications for the coming physician surplus. *Journal of Health and Social Behavior, 26,* 297–311.

Salloway, J. C. (1982). *Health care delivery systems.* Boulder, CO: Westview Publishing.

Sammons, J. H. (1989). Physician payment reform: Don't forget the patient. *Health Affairs, 8,* 132–137.

Shapiro, E., & Tate, R. B. (1989). Is health care changing? A comparison between physician, hospital, nursing home, and home care use of two elderly cohorts. *Medical Care, 27,* 1002–1014.

Stoeckle, J. D. (1987). Working on the factory floor. *Annals of Internal Medicine, 107,* 250–251.

Stoeckle, J. D. (1988). Reflections on modern doctoring. *The Milbank Quarterly, 66,* S76–S91.

Tobin, S. (1977). *Effective social services for older Americans.* Detroit: Wayne State Gerontology Center.

Twaddle, A., & Hessler, R. (1987). *A sociology of health* (2nd ed.). New York: MacMillan.

Verbrugge, L. M. (1984). Longer life but worsening health: Trends in health and mortality of middle-aged and older women. *Milbank Memorial Fund Quarterly, 62,* 475–519.

Waitzkin, H. (1989). A critical theory of medical discourse: Ideology, social control, and the processing of social context in medical encounters. *Journal of Health and Social Behavior, 30,* 220–239.

Ward, R. (1978). Services for older people: An integrated framework for research. *Journal of Health and Social Behavior, 18,* 61–70.

Weinstein, M. C., & Stason, W. B. (1985). Cost-effectiveness of interventions to prevent or treat coronary heart disease. *Annual Review of Public Health, 6,* 41–63.

West, C. (1984). *Routine complications: Troubles with talk between doctors and patients.* Bloomington: Indiana University Press.

Whisnant, J. P. (1984). The decline of stroke. *Stroke, 15,* 160–168.

Wolinsky, F. D. (1988a). *The sociology of health: Principles, practitioners, and issues* (2nd ed.). Belmont: Wadsworth.

Wolinsky, F. D. (1988b). The professional dominance perspective, revisited. *The Milbank Quarterly, 66,* S33–S47.

Wolinsky, F. D., Aguirre, B. E., Fann, L. J., Keith, V. M., Arnold, C. L., Niederhauer, J., & Dietrich, K. (1989). Ethnic differences in the demand for physician and hospital utilization: Conspicuous evidence of considerable inequalities. *Milbank Quarterly, 67,* 412–449.

Wolinsky, F. D., & Arnold, C. L. (1989). A birth cohort analysis of dental contact among elderly Americans. *American Journal of Public Health, 79,* 47–51.

Wolinsky, F. D., & Coe, R. M. (1984). Physician and hospital utilization among elderly adults: An analysis of the health interview survey. *Journal of Gerontology, 39,* 334–341.

Wolinsky, F. D., Coe, R. M., Chavez, M. N., Prendergast, J. M., & Miller, D. K.

(1986). Further assessment of the reliability and validity of a nutritional risk index: Analysis of a three-wave panel study of elderly adults. *Health Services Research, 20,* 977–990.

Wolinsky, F. D., Coe, R. M., & Mosely, R. R. (1987). The use of health services by elderly Americans: Implications from a regression-based cohort analysis. In R. Ward & S. Tobin (Eds.), *Health in aging: Sociological issues and policy directions* (pp. 106–132). New York: Springer.

Wolinsky, F. D., Mosely, R. R., & Coe, R. M. (1986). A cohort analysis of the use of health services by elderly Americans. *Journal of Health and Social Behavior, 27,* 209–219.

Index

158363